Polarity Thinking in Healthcare: The Missing Logic to Achieve Transformation

Bonnie Wesorick

HRD Press, Inc. ● Amherst, Massachusetts

Polarity Thinking™, Polarity Management™, and Polarity Map™ are registered trademarks of Barry Johnson and Polarity Partnerships, LLC (www.polaritypartnership.com). Used with permission.

Published by: HRD Press, Inc.
22 Amherst Road
Amherst, MA 01002
413-253-3488
800-822-2801 (U.S. and Canada)
413-253-3490 (fax)
www.hrdpress.com

ISBN 978-1-61014-406-3

Editorial services by Sally M. Farnham
Production services by Jean Miller
Cover design by Eileen Klockars

Table of Contents

Foreword

Bonnie and I have been fellow travelers for 20 years. We have been learning from each other about how to apply Polarity Thinking™ to healthcare, and her vision and passion are contagious. She has been a tireless advocate for both those who deliver healthcare and those who receive it, and it is this dual focus that is the underlying polarity for her new book. She understands the importance of these interdependent pairs of values, from their basic principles to their application in every aspect of a healthcare system. Bonnie knows healthcare "from the bedside out."

I do not know enough about healthcare management to write this book for healthcare professionals, so I am extremely grateful that Bonnie is bringing our shared learning about polarities to you and your care-giving colleagues. You are in for a treat. My hope is that you will be interested enough to go beyond reading this book and join Bonnie and a growing community of other healthcare professionals who use Polarity Thinking in their own clinical settings—and experience the benefits.

Barry Johnson
Organizational Development consultant
and creator of the Polarity Thinking™ Approach

Dedication

This book is dedicated to my husband, David Dell Wesorick, who has inspired me, supported me, and most importantly helped me leverage the many polarities of life. Together, we have experienced a quality of life that neither of us could have achieved alone.

Preface

When I stepped into the world of healthcare in 1961, I was a student nurse, surrounded by committed, intelligent people. When I entered into practice, it was the daily realities, both good and bad, that launched me into my then and present life's work: to co-create the best places to give and receive care. I noticed that many healthcare providers spent more waking hours at work than they did in their own homes. The need for these healers of our humanity to have healthy cultures and supports to deliver their care was apparent. I was driven by a deep passion to help create a healthcare system worthy of the commitment of the healers and a system deserving of our patients' trust.

Initially, I had no idea how challenging it would be to carry out the logical and obvious work necessary to make a difference for those who give and who receive care. The culture was hierarchical, task-dominated, often margin-driven, and fragmented because of the lack of coordination and integration of care across disciplines and settings. Institutional and professional barriers were evident. People were not clear about accountabilities and ways to carry out their responsibilities in partnerships with teams made up of caregivers and patients. I also did not understand the resistance. I was looking for a realistic goal to set and a place to start.

I searched for professionals who had led change efforts, and I read everything I could. I remember being influenced by the wisdom of many, but I was struck by the warning of Florence Nightingale: "The world, more especially this hospital world, is in such a hurry, moving so fast that it is too easy to slide into bad habits before we are aware."

She wrote those words over 150 years ago, but they are today's realities. Florence Nightingale was warning of the dangers that led to the very realities surrounding me: a hierarchical culture and a task-dominated, institutionalized, and fragmented system of care.

Why in over 150 years have we not been able to solve some obvious problems? Why in a profession attracting the most intelligent, committed people in the world were so many of the same problems surfacing over and over again and not going away? Was it because no one noticed? Or that we just could not figure out the answer? That did not make sense, because I was surrounded by advancements in so many other areas of healthcare. Who would have thought back in 1961 that we would be replacing body parts? What did we need to learn or know before this cycle could be changed?

I thought I had figured it out. We simply need to change from the old ways of thinking to a new way of thinking. I even wrote a book about it titled: *The Closing and Opening of a Millennium: A Journey from Old to New Thinking.* The message of the book was that we need to shift from old to new ways of thinking in order to remove the barriers—barriers that were holding us back—to improve practice and culture. I started to name the old and new paradigms and talked of the impact they had on our cultures and practice. I listed the many paradigms in pairs of old and new, such as institutional service to professional service; medical care model to healthcare model; mechanistic to dynamic connectedness; cost of care to quality of care; dependent to independent; and limited strategies to endless possibilities.

As I drew the diagrams showing the shift from old to new paradigms, I became aware that something was not right. The assumption around paradigms is ***moving from one to another.*** It is letting go of one way of thinking and replacing it with another. That didn't work because what I called a "new" paradigm did not replace the familiar old paradigm. I remember being challenged by a seasoned, excellent nurse clinician—a master of institutional services—who did not believe we should be replacing everything, including what was working well. "It is not about giving up institutional services," she explained. "I know they are essential." She was right: institutional and professional services were and are equally important. I realized that there was no model to connect what I called an old paradigm and a new paradigm. She helped me realize that my way of thinking was incomplete: *Is this missing piece of logic the reason why we hadn't been able to fix some of the major issues facing healthcare even with the best minds?* I asked myself: *What is this missing link?*

The search for the missing link led me to Barry Johnson, a seasoned organizational development professional who has dedicated his academic and professional life to sharing a model he created that describes the missing logic. It is called Polarity Thinking. I studied it and asked many questions about its effectiveness, and then I realized that I had found *the missing link.*

I started using the Polarity Thinking Model and began to introduce it to healthcare colleagues. I explained why the same problems kept surfacing over and over again and why we have not been able to reach or sustain new possibilities. I was now able to share how the model can be used to break this cycle and improve our cultures and practice.

I watched clinicians get excited and heard the "aha's." Colleagues shared feelings of relief and hope that many of the problems that were draining their energy and keeping them awake at night could now be addressed. They wanted to know more and seemed eager to learn how to integrate it with their daily responsibilities and bring it to others.

It is this experience that has driven me to write this book and bring this new way of thinking, the missing logic, to all who are committed to the health of others. We are the healers for this humanity, and it is my hope that it will give you a wisdom that enhances all aspects of *your* work and life.

Introduction

The purpose of this book is to help you and other healthcare leaders achieve the vision to create a quality, integrated, cost-effective healthcare system that supports the wellbeing of humanity. Author Max DePree says to achieve any vision, the first responsibility of a leader is to define reality. When reality is accurately defined, the nature of the transformation work that bridges the gap from reality to the desired vision becomes transparent. Polarity Thinking (PT) provides an additional lens to help one define reality. The focus of this book will be at the point-of-care, the place where the hands of those who *give* care and the hands of those who *receive* care meet.

Our colleagues on the front lines are tired of new programs and projects that work for a while yet are not sustainable over time. Each change effort starts off with good intentions but ends up with the same old problems surfacing over and over again. Despite our having the most advanced medical care in the world, we are living within a work culture that is plagued with dissatisfaction and discouragement. There are shortages: not just in money but also healthcare professionals. Those who dedicate their lives to caring for this humanity lose heart in dehumanized, fragmented environments where workloads are constantly increasing. People feel alone, powerless, and voiceless in the midst of the demands. Some experience an exhaustion that no day off or extra hours of sleep will make go away.

It is time to break this cycle. Polarity Thinking has helped hundreds do just that, and it will help you.

This book is divided into three sections.

Section One: Chapters 1 through 13 are devoted to introducing and explaining the basic principles of Polarity Thinking. It begins with knowing what polarities look like and how they work. Since we are, and must be, strong problem solvers, it is important to know how this skill impacts our ability to understand and leverage or manage polarities. Each chapter in this section will build on the basics and deepen your understanding of Polarity Thinking by relating the principles to *your* everyday realities. The polarities presented are prioritized based on the lessons learned from over 400 rural, community, and university settings in North America, members of the Clinical Practice Model Resource Center's (CPMRC) International Consortium. Once polarities are understood, it is natural to ask, "How do we know if we are leveraging or managing them well?" A process for evaluation will be reviewed.

Section Two: Six interdependent pairs of values (polarities) that are at the heart of the transformational work will be reviewed. These additional polarities, fundamental to creating the best places to give and receive care, build on the polarities discussed in the chapters.

Section Three: A summary of the principles of Polarity Thinking, tips, and strategies presented throughout the book.

Each section will highlight some of the lessons learned by our consortium partners. The nature of their collective work to transform cultures and practice at the point-of-care has uncovered common polarities that are essential to leverage in order to create the best places to give and receive care. The experience and wisdom of our partners are reflected throughout this book.

Additional information, including a selected bibliography, appears in the back.

Section One:
Principles of Polarity Thinking

Chapter 1
The Missing Logic

"The greatest danger in times of turbulence is not the turbulence; it is to act with yesterday's logic."

— Peter Drucker

Our lives and our work as healthcare professionals are too important to be controlled by poor decisions, quick fixes, unintended consequences, and reactionary responses to ever-changing external events, statistics, fads, and fear (our own and that of others). Leaders are as responsible for making accurate diagnoses of reality as clinicians are for making accurate diagnoses for the people they care for. It is time to learn new skills that help us think, serve, and relate together to create a healthy, integrated work culture and healthcare system.

The next few chapters will focus on how to use Polarity Thinking in healthcare settings, *where the hands of those who give care and the hands of those who receive care meet.*

Polarities and Polarity Thinking

Polarity Thinking provides insights into complex situations, giving hope and direction to improve reality.

So what is Polarity Thinking?

It is a way of thinking that helps one understand the difference between problems to solve and polarities that need to be leveraged. It includes a principle driven model to leverage polarities. The formal systematic approach provides a framework that leads to levels of clarity not previously achieved by old ways of thinking. It is the missing logic that can be used to reach new outcomes and possibilities needed to advance our cultures and our practices.

What are polarities?

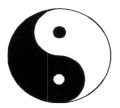

Do you recognize this symbol? People who are asked to identify it generally respond correctly: yin and yang, the Chinese symbol representing two complementary forces that work better together than they do apart. They know that it is an ancient symbol, but it is only when they talk about it that they begin to use words that define a polarity.

What is a polarity? The working definition for *polarity* that we will be using in this book is: an interdependent pair of values or alternative points of view that appear different and unrelated, competitive, or even opposite, but in reality need each other over time to reach outcomes neither can reach alone.

They are often thought of as dilemmas or paradoxes. They are present in our daily lives and in every important problem and every important decision. Just as gravity is a natural, predictable phenomenon, so are polarities.

If you are unfamiliar with Polarity Thinking, you will find yourself misdiagnosing critical situations. The ramifications are predictable and most assuredly will lead to unintended consequences and destructive outcomes similar to that from any natural phenomena. For example, being unaware of spontaneous combustion can lead to fires within haylofts in barns. This natural phenomenon does not happen right away but will *over time.* We can avoid unintended consequences over time by understanding and using the principles of Polarity Thinking.

A Clinical Scenario:

If I were asked to name one of the priority polarities that every hospital must leverage, it would be *mission* (the quality of care) and *margin* (the cost of care). I had the opportunity to provide a workshop related to the transformational work of creating best places to give and receive care at two different large (800–1,000 beds) urban hospitals, one in Canada and one in the United States. Both were experiencing financial challenges. Neither group was familiar with the concept of polarities. I carried out the same exercise at each hospital: I asked each individual leader to pick either mission or margin as their preferred pole. If they picked mission, they stood on the right side of the room; if they picked margin, they stood on the left side of the room.

At both hospitals, something happened that I had never seen in all my years of doing this activity: at one place, all the leaders were standing on the mission side, and at the other place, all the leaders were standing on the margin side! With polarities, this is an ominous sign. You will understand what I mean by this as you read on. By the end of this chapter, you will undoubtedly have some thoughts about this unusual occurrence.

**Illusion developed by Danish psychologist
Edgar Rubin (1886–1951)**

Edgar Rubin's now famous illusion represents a paradox, similar in concept to the polarities discussed in this chapter. When you look at the illustration, what do you immediately see? Some people see two faces in profile right away, while others will see a vase. The illusion tells us that an individual's perception is an intimate and important part of the whole. However, if you see only one image, such as the profiles, you see only half of what is there! It is hard to define reality if you see only half of the truth.

The figure is a good example of two very different "objects"—two sides of a face, and a vase. For the purposes of understanding the entire illustration, we can call it an **interdependent pair,** ***because both are working together to create the whole.*** If you take away the profiles in white, you will also lose the vase. If you take away the black vase, you will lose the two profiles. The black parts and the white parts need each other to create something neither can do alone. This is an important principle that helps explain polarities.

Polarities help us see the whole of reality, and both poles of a polarity together create something more complete. Polarities are present in every problem you encounter as a leader in healthcare—problems that keep us awake at night, such as patient and staff safety, mission and margin stability, fragmentation, duplication, repetition, inconsistent patient care, and the stress of increasing demands and expectations from professional, governmental, and credentialing organizations—with minimal reimbursement.

Why do these chronic issues never seem to go away for good, despite great efforts to address them? Why do so many problems get fixed and then return with a vengeance? Why in a system filled with intelligent, committed, caring professionals are there so many who are tired, overworked, taken for granted, and discouraged with their work culture? These problems are chronic: all the problem-solving approaches, no matter how good or how costly, will not make some problems go away permanently.

Why not? Because many of these chronic situations are misdiagnosed as problems to be solved, when in fact, they are just polarities that need to be leveraged and managed.

In my work, I have come to learn that great leaders who have broad experience and intuition already know about polarities, and their organizations reap the benefits of this wisdom. However, this wisdom is often tacit. In order to increase innovation and more readily reach sustainable outcomes, leaders need to not only understand polarities, but also understand that this way of thinking—this missing logic—needs to become as common as the skill of problem solving. Understanding polarities offers a new level of thinking. *When leaders misdiagnose a polarity for a problem, those who give and receive care experience unintended negative consequences. When leaders are not clear about how to differentiate between problems and polarities, there is wasted time, money, and energy.*

We can no longer pretend that all is well when it is not. Equally important, we must not assume that all is hopeless. ***We have so many possibilities!*** Leveraging and managing polarities will enable us to reach many possibilities that cannot be reached by problem solving alone. Many of the clinical organizations I have studied and worked with were reenergized when they experienced the possibilities inherent when problem solving is supplemented with Polarity Thinking.

I have seen so many success stories in my work, and I will share some of their experiences throughout the remaining chapters. Diane Humbrecht, Chief Nursing Informatics Officer, DNP, RN, at Abington Health in Abington, Pennsylvania, leads point-of-care transformation and passed on some helpful insights:

> "Polarity Thinking is a great tool to lean on when you are attempting to hard-wire complex change. It allows for clarity of purpose to emerge, and engages those responsible for the 'work' to see how their efforts contribute to success. Polarity Thinking is my 'go to' process when I'm stuck and don't seem to be able to sustain change. Often the analysis phase of problem solving is either very short or eliminated as we jump directly to solutions without fully understanding the tension of the competing priorities and how each contributes not only to the complexity of the issue at hand, but also to the nature of the solutions."

Diane has addressed the many polarities inherent in the work of transformation at the bedside. When she and colleagues were able to manage polarities, the following possibilities became reality. The Abington Health team experienced the following:

- rapid achievement of desired outcomes
- automation but not dehumanization
- fiscal soundness without decreasing quality
- standardization without interfering with new ideas
- evidence-based patient care without losing individualized care
- enhanced interprofessional partnerships across the continuum of care without losing individual identity
- the completion of basic tasks without decreasing professional scope of practice
- the provision of medical treatment without losing preventive care
- innovation without losing stability
- improved productivity without losing human sensitivity
- clinical integration without decreasing productivity
- implementation of integrated documentation without resistance
- decrease variability of care without being rigid

It is important to know that polarities never go away and cannot be solved, but hold all the possibilities listed above when they are leveraged. The next chapter will help you understand the approach to those possibilities.

Chapter 2

What Polarities Look Like and How They Work

"The soul never thinks without a picture."

— Aristotle

A seasoned, respected physician decided to get his MBA. He prided himself on being a continuous learner and one who was open to new and different ways of thinking. As a director of an acute care department, he was well aware of the clinical realities, the need for change to address the safety problems, and the work to sustain a healthy culture. He realized that the healthcare system was in need of change.

He wondered what it would take to actually achieve the changes. He said he felt that leaders needed to be courageous, and he was not sure he had that courage. He knew how hard it was to show someone that their thinking was not correct. Following an introduction to Polarity Thinking in his MBA class, he said he was relieved and that understanding polarities gave him courage because he could start off with You are right and I am right, but we are both only half right.

The Polarity Thinking approach was developed by organizational design consultant Barry Johnson over two decades ago. Johnson believed that if the principles of Polarity Thinking could be visualized on paper, it would deepen individual understanding and help people enhance the skill of leveraging and managing polarities. He developed a structure called the Polarity Map™ that records the *principles and dynamics* of all interdependent pairs. Johnson and his colleagues laid out a process having five components or steps (Seeing, Mapping, Assessing, Learning, and Leveraging) that explains the principles and process of addressing polarities. This chapter will focus on the information you need to know about the principles of Polarity Thinking. This first step will also appear as part of the additional examples in the remaining chapters.

Polarity Thinking: An Overview

The Polarity Thinking approach begins with the concept of interrelated pairs of values inherent in a problem or situation that are equal in value and must work together in order to create a more powerful whole. They must each be leveraged or managed. The step-by-step process itself is best understood by organizing the components on a four-quadrant grid so that the individuals using the approach can see the advantages and disadvantages of each part of the pair and hence maximize their strengths to mutual advantage.

The Basic Polarity Map appears on the following page. There are 11 components to the map. As we work through this section, you will see that each part is important to the step-by-step process to leverage each polarity.

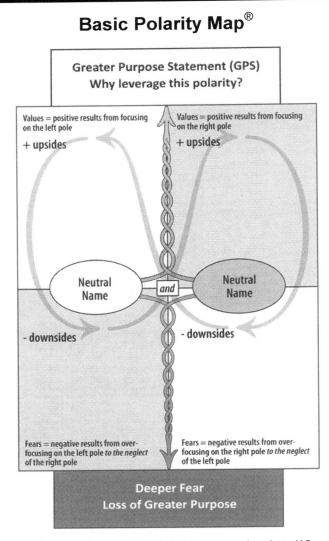

Basic Polarity Map®

Greater Purpose Statement (GPS)
Why leverage this polarity?

Values = positive results from focusing on the left pole

+ upsides

Values = positive results from focusing on the right pole

+ upsides

Neutral Name   *and*   Neutral Name

- downsides

- downsides

Fears = negative results from over-focusing on the left pole *to the neglect* of the right pole

Fears = negative results from over-focusing on the right pole *to the neglect* of the left pole

Deeper Fear
Loss of Greater Purpose

Polarity Map © 1992, 2008 Polarity Management Associates, LLC

The eleven components of the Basic Polarity Map:

1–2. **An interdependent pair:** Placement for the names of each pole of the interdependent pair.

3. **The infinity loop:** The loop visualizes the natural tension/energy around each pole.

4. **Greater purpose statement (GPS):** A goal or outcome that neither pole can "reach" alone. It answers the question *Why leverage this polarity?*

5. **Greater fear:** The failure to achieve greater purpose if action is not taken to support one or both poles.

6. **Virtuous cycle:** This arrow shows that tension/energy is moving toward the greater purpose.

7. **Vicious cycle:** This arrow shows that the tension/energy is moving toward the greater fear.

8–9. **Upside quadrants (2):** These spaces are reserved for the lists of positive/upside outcomes (one for each pole).

10–11. **Downside quadrants (2):** These spaces are reserved for the lists of negative/downside outcomes (one for each pole).

As you identify and place each component in its respective position on the map, you will come to understand the fundamental principles of Polarity Thinking.

Here are the main components as they would appear on a polarity map:

1. **The Interdependent Pair and Its Two Poles**

   The mapping process begins with the ellipses that represent each part of an interdependent pair (alternative values or points of view).

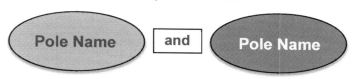

The names of the poles, such as Mission and Margin, are placed in the ellipses. It is important that each pole be given a "neutral" name, because there is no one positive pole and there is no one negative pole. *Both* are equally important.

2. **The Infinity Loop**

   The infinity loop visualizes the movement of the natural tension/energy that exists between each pole.

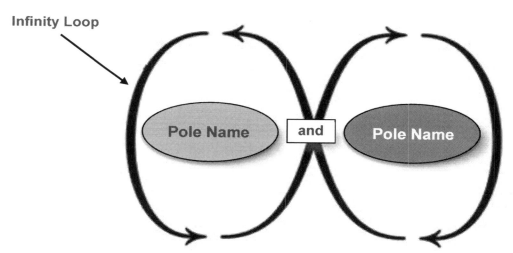

Each pole is different and represents an alternative view, so there will always be tension/energy between them. The good news is that *this tension can be leveraged.* The infinity loop shows the flow of tension/energy around each pole and its movement from one pole to the other via the arrows.

The infinity loop is a visualization of where the tension is between the poles.

3. **Additional Components of the Basic Polarity Map**

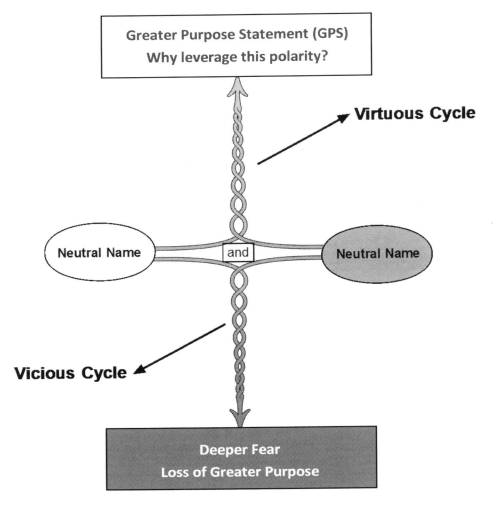

The box at the top shows the greater purpose statement (GPS). It is a goal that can only be reached if both poles are interdependently supported and the tension between them creates a virtuous cycle that leads to a greater purpose, a goal that neither pole can reach alone.

The box at the bottom shows the deeper fear when the tension between the two poles is not leveraged and it moves in a vicious cycle toward the deeper fear, the opposite or loss of the greater purpose.

4. **The Visualization of the Movement of the Tension Represented by the Infinity Loop between the Poles**

   A. **Tension Being Leveraged:**

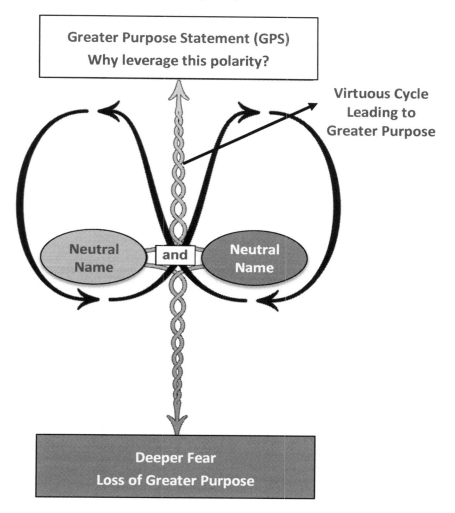

Visualization of Outcomes when Tension is Leveraged
Basic Polarity Map®

The above illustration shows what the infinity loop looks like when action steps are being taken to leverage the tension and support of both poles in order to reach the greater purpose.

B. **Tension Not Being Leveraged:**

The illustration below is showing what the infinity loop looks like when action steps are not being taken to leverage the tension that exists around both poles and the tension moves to the deeper fear.

Visualization of Outcomes when Tension is Not Leveraged

Basic Polarity Map®

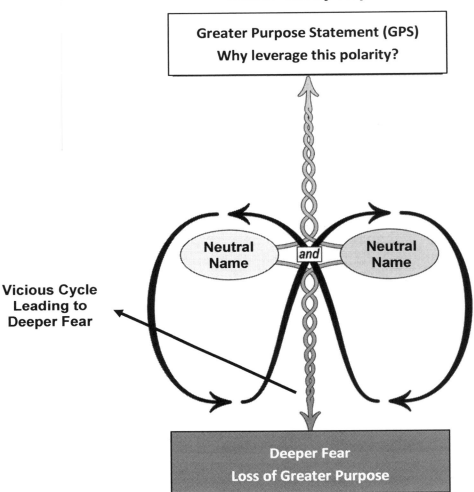

5. **The Four Quadrants Complete the Basic Polarity Map**

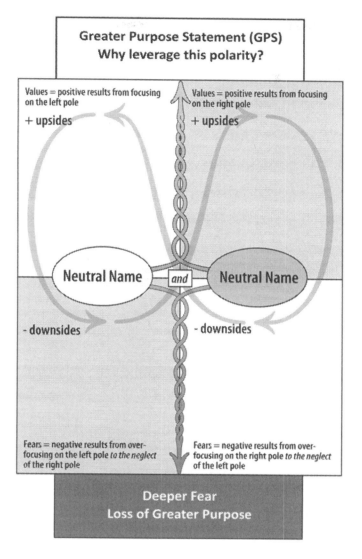

This figure shows the finished Basic Map by placing four shaded quadrants that are "placeholders" for the description of the positive (upsides) and the negative (downsides) of each pole. The quadrant components of the map are a place for the second step in the SMALL process; that is, the "M" for mapping or placing the content specific to the polarity within the map.

How do the components work together?

The mapping process can be used in any real-life situation where there are two competing values that need to work together for maximum effectiveness and how they can be easily leveraged. The use of a metaphor will increase the clarity of each component of the map and deepen the understanding of the principles of Polarity Thinking. The very familiar physiological metaphor of breathing provides an introductory process and makes the key principles of the Basic Map come alive.

Let's fill in the content for each part of the map, using the breathing metaphor.

Inhale and Exhale

Basic Polarity Map®

Greater Purpose Statement (GPS)
Live
Why leverage this polarity?

Values = positive results from focusing on the left pole

+ upsides

Increased Oxygen

Inhale

and

Values = positive results from focusing on the right pole

+ upsides

Decreased Carbon Dioxide

Exhale

- downsides

Increased Carbon Dioxide

- downsides

Decreased Oxygen

Fears = negative results from over-focusing on the left pole *to the neglect* of the right pole

Fears = negative results from over-focusing on the right pole *to the neglect* of the left pole

Deeper Fear
Die
Loss of Greater Purpose

With this metaphor, we have two logical poles with neutral names: Inhale and Exhale. Remember, one pole is not positive and the other negative—each represents important positive values or outcomes, despite their different properties. This is true of all polarities. We reserve places on the map for this information: The positive quadrants reflect the value or desired outcomes associated with each pole of Inhale and Exhale. They are referred to as the upside of the pole. There are also quadrants for the negative content (with feared outcomes). These quadrants are referred to as downsides.

The upside of the Inhale pole when we perform the action is that our body gets more oxygen ("increase oxygen"). The upside of the Exhale pole is that we lower the levels of carbon dioxide ("decrease carbon dioxide"). In order to live, we need both—one is not more important than the other.

Now look at the arrows: The virtuous or vertical arrow between the upper quadrants for the poles shows us that if we can inhale as well as exhale, we will live. To live is our goal—our greater purpose. Obviously, it is *a goal neither pole can reach alone*.

The inhale/exhale metaphor provides a way to experience the dynamics of the infinity loop. The principles come alive in the following exercise.

Exercise: The Infinity Loop

Take a very slow deep breath over 15 seconds and hold it. As you begin the continuous slow deep breath, it feels good. You are getting O^2 building up in your body, which is the positive value of the Inhale pole.

But what happens *over time?* You feel tension and are beginning to experience the downside of Inhale—an increase in carbon dioxide. The tension you are feeling is a reminder to exhale and get rid of the CO^2 building up in your body, which is the positive value of the Exhale pole. This is an important principle because it helps you experience or feel the need for oscillation from one pole to the other.

The natural flow of the tension/energy between the two poles is necessary to achieve the upside of both poles. This oscillation is represented by the infinity loop. The positive movement of that tension supports the virtuous cycle arrow, which leads to the greater purpose statement that neither pole can reach alone.

Each pole has two parts: positive outcomes, and fear of the loss of the positive outcomes. These are placed in diagonal quadrants.

Basic Polarity Map®

Greater Purpose Statement (GPS)
Live
Why leverage this polarity?

Values = positive results from focusing on the left pole

+ upsides

Values = positive results from focusing on the right pole

+ upsides

Increased Oxygen

Inhale *and* Exhale

- downsides

- downsides

Decreased Oxygen

Fears = negative results from over-focusing on the left pole *to the neglect* of the right pole

Fears = negative results from over-focusing on the right pole *to the neglect* of the left pole

Deeper Fear
Die
Loss of Greater Purpose

The Basic Map makes visible the relationship between interdependent poles. The above illustration highlights that each pole represents two parts of the map: the positive values of the pole and the fear of loss of the positive values. Note how this fact is represented on the map. The positive for inhale is in the upper left quadrant and the fear of its loss is in the right lower diagonal quadrant. *The diagonals reflect this reality and it is true for all polarities.*

The Infinity Loop

The infinity loop visualizes the consequences if one pole is neglected in favor of the other.

Basic Polarity Map®

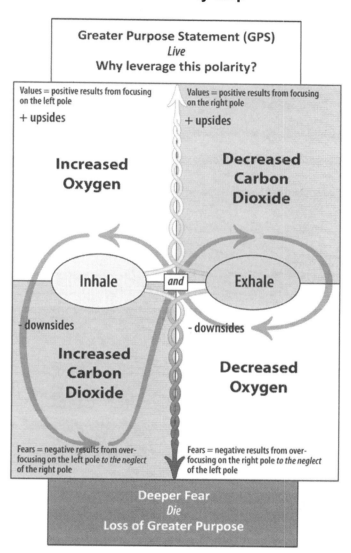

Every interdependent value or point of view on its own, over time, will produce negative outcomes—what we refer to here as a *downside.* If you chose to only inhale, you will soon experience the **downside** of the Inhale pole, resulting in an increased level of CO^2, as seen in the illustration above showing the infinity loop moving to the downside of Inhale.

The infinity loop visualizes the consequences if one pole is neglected in favor of the other.

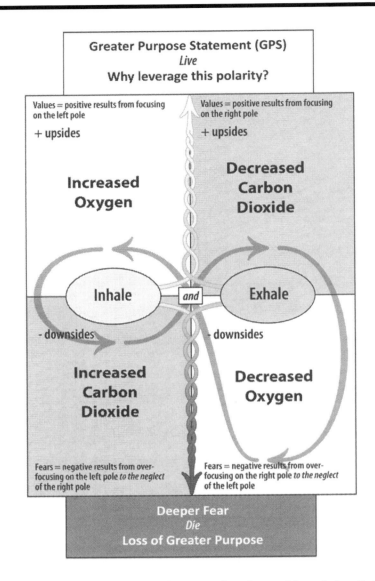

Greater Purpose Statement (GPS)
Live
Why leverage this polarity?

Values = positive results from focusing on the left pole

+ upsides

Values = positive results from focusing on the right pole

+ upsides

Increased Oxygen

Decreased Carbon Dioxide

Inhale *and* Exhale

- downsides

- downsides

Increased Carbon Dioxide

Decreased Oxygen

Fears = negative results from over-focusing on the left pole *to the neglect* of the right pole

Fears = negative results from over-focusing on the right pole *to the neglect* of the left pole

Deeper Fear
Die
Loss of Greater Purpose

If you choose only to exhale, you will experience the **downside** of the Exhale pole, resulting in decreased oxygen. As seen in the illustration above, the infinity loop moves to the downside of Exhale. Whenever you choose to focus on only one pole and essentially neglect the other, you create a **vicious downward spiral**. This negative momentum is seen by the spiral arrow, which ultimately leads to the **greater fear/concern** or the opposite of the **greater purpose.** In this case, that is death.

The inhale/exhale metaphor makes it very clear that when you have interdependent values, it is *a waste of time* to argue which pole is more important. It is not black or white, or a choice between one or the other. Neither pole is a sustainable solution, because there is no problem to be solved here. The poles are interdependent and *both must exist* and be supported. If you choose one over the other, you will always lose (in our example here, you *will* die). You cannot fix the inhale/exhale issue, because *it is ongoing and can never be solved.* One pole is not the problem and the other a solution; if Exhale was a solution, then once we exhaled, the breathing problem would be fixed. However, it isn't solved at all— *the oscillation between both poles is absolutely essential.* Now let's look at the role of tension.

Self-Correcting Movement of Tension

Basic Polarity Map®

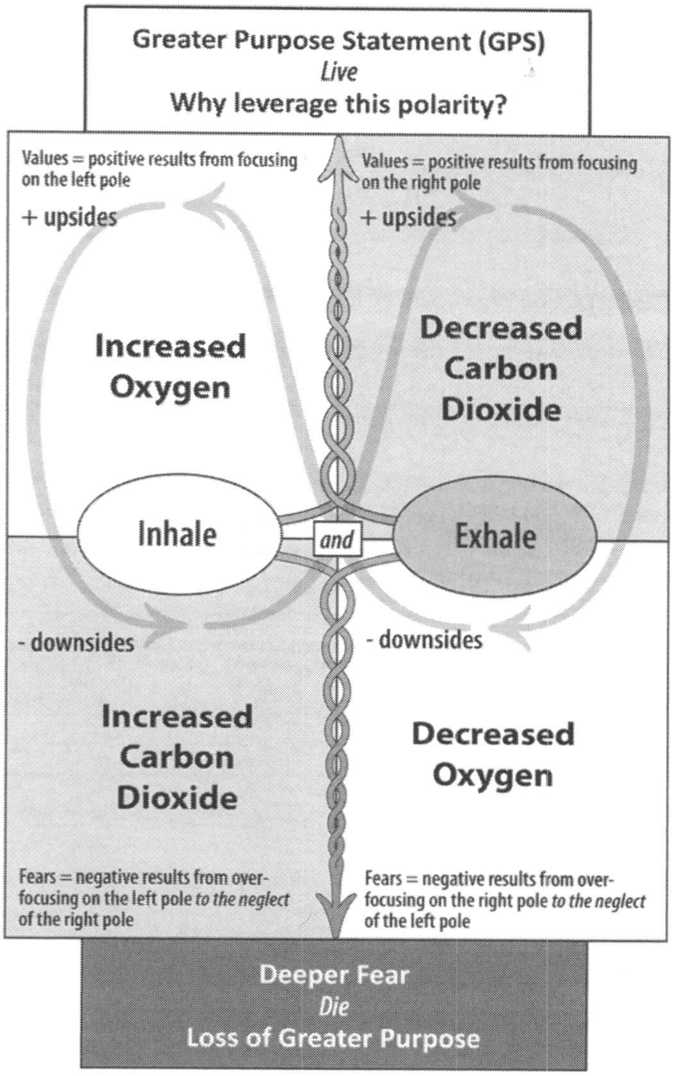

Greater Purpose Statement (GPS)
Live
Why leverage this polarity?

Values = positive results from focusing on the left pole

+ upsides

Increased Oxygen

Values = positive results from focusing on the right pole

+ upsides

Decreased Carbon Dioxide

Inhale *and* Exhale

- downsides

Increased Carbon Dioxide

- downsides

Decreased Oxygen

Fears = negative results from over-focusing on the left pole *to the neglect* of the right pole

Fears = negative results from over-focusing on the right pole *to the neglect* of the left pole

Deeper Fear
Die
Loss of Greater Purpose

To reach our goal, we need to leverage the tension. The movement of tension/energy—the oscillation between the poles—is represented by the infinity loop in the illustration above.

Do you remember riding a teeter totter when you were little? If you do, you no doubt remember what happens if you are on the upside and your friend suddenly jumps off. You fall to the ground.

That is what happens when polarities are treated as problems to be solved: the bottom will drop out. Without oscillation in breathing, the individual simply dies. No goal was achieved. The oscillation in a well-leveraged and managed polarity moves between the upper positive quadrants. *The tension you felt with the breathing exercise is present in all polarities and explains the movement between the upper quadrants that is driven by anticipating or experiencing the downside of one pole combined with the attraction to the upside of the other pole.* Look again at the illustration above. Can you see the self-correcting movement pictured there? It is necessary if you want to manage or leverage polarities.

The inhale/exhale metaphor demonstrates the underlying principles of polarities. The fact that both poles are equally important is easier to accept in the inhale/exhale metaphor than it might be in other polarities. With most of the dilemmas that haunt healthcare providers, the downsides of a specific value (pole) are not obvious, certainly not within seconds or minutes like those in the breathing metaphor.

Most negative consequences or downsides are not even noticed until a longer period of time has elapsed and the situation reaches a critical stage. People seem to become so focused on improving or strengthening one value and do not realize that they are neglecting its interdependent value (pole). They develop a false sense of security and truly believe that they are on the right track using the typical problem-solving mindset that got them into trouble in the first place.

Moving from Metaphor to Reality at a Personal Level

There are many different types of interdependent pairs in nature and in all the areas of our lives (personal, professional organizational, global and universal community). There are also different kinds of polarities: **intrinsic** to life such as the Inhale/Exhale polarity and **chosen** such as the Work and Home polarity. If you do not work, then obviously this is not a polarity you need to leverage.

The focus of this book is to show how Polarity Thinking is used in healthcare. The principles of this approach are generally introduced gradually by first applying them to a familiar and/or personal polarity that we must manage day-to-day, for example, the Work and Home polarity. The quality of your life is determined by how well you are able to make the most of each part of the interdependent pair so that what you achieve by getting the two to work interdependently is far greater than if you strengthened only one and virtually ignored the other.

The Work and Home polarity is a good one to start with, because most of us have experienced the upsides and the downsides of each pole and know it is an ongoing situation.

With most polarities, people seem to show a preference for one pole over the other, often without realizing it. However, most of us feel strongly about both Work and Home, so this pair is especially useful in emphasizing the need *not* to choose one or the other when it comes to leveraging. With other polarities that will be discussed in this book, valuing both poles is not as obvious or as easy as this one. That is why this polarity is a good one to begin with.

Before a polarity can be leveraged, we need to start the mapping process by first identifying the positive values (upsides) and the negative concerns (downsides) for each pole and then filling in the content of each part of the map. Work and Home each have strong positive values, as well as equally important downsides (consequences if one pole is neglected). Filling in the content of a map is always a values and language clarification process. It is critical that the words used to describe the values or fears/concerns listed on the map in each pole reflect the individual's or the group's own words.

Filling in the map requires one to ask some important questions:

1. What are the positive outcomes of each pole?

2. What are the negative outcomes or the loss of each pole's upside if one pole is neglected (the diagonals on the map)?

3. What is the greater purpose statement that can be reached if both poles are supported or leveraged?

4. What is the deeper fear/concern of not leveraging this polarity well?

Exercise: Creating a Personal Map

Before you fill in each section of the Work and Home polarity map shown below, reflect on your values related to the questions on page 22 and make a note of them.

Work and Home Polarity Map

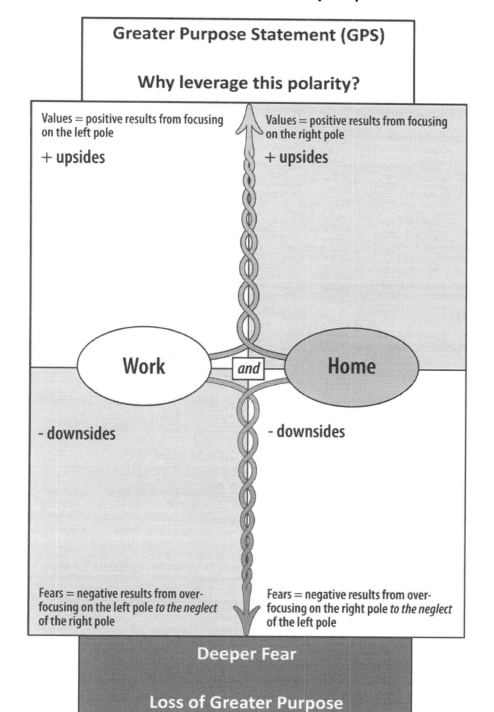

Exercise: Creating a Personal Map (continued)

1. **Fill in the map on the previous page, using your own words.** Start by filling in the upsides of the pole that you have the stronger preference for. (Remember: There is no right or wrong feeling here—both are important. However, it is good to know which one you are more drawn to.)

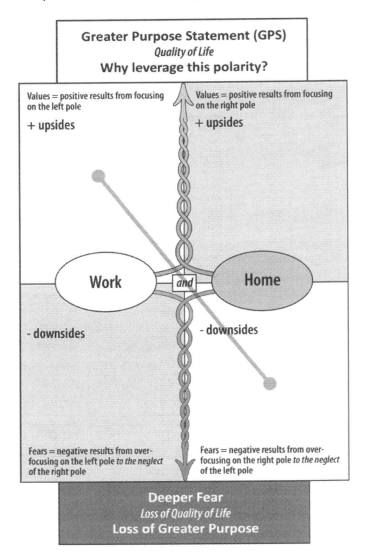

Diagonal Quadrants

When you have a preference for one pole, you often have concerns or fear about the downside of the other pole because it represents a loss of some things you value about your preference pole (diagonal quadrants, as seen in the illustration above). Because you have the upside of this pole filled in, you know what to put in the diagonal: the loss of those very things you value about your preference.

2. **Fill in the upside of the other pole.** That may not be as easy as filling in the upside of your preference pole, but when you do it, you will have the information that makes transparent the downside of your preference pole. **Note:** *Sometimes it is hard to fill in the downside of the preference pole because we are often blind to the downside of the pole we prefer.* It is important to remember that the downside of one's preference pole is usually more difficult to describe. Often we are unaware of the impact or downside of our preference pole—especially when it comes to the effects it has on others who might have to "live with the consequences because you did not leverage both poles".

3. **Fill in the greater purpose statement.** When the upsides of Work and the upsides of Home are both strong, what will be the outcome? A common greater purpose statement is to achieve "quality of life." If Work is strong but Home is not, or vice versa, the "quality of life" is decreased. Fill in the deeper fear—the loss of your greater purpose.

Completed Map for Work and Home Polarity

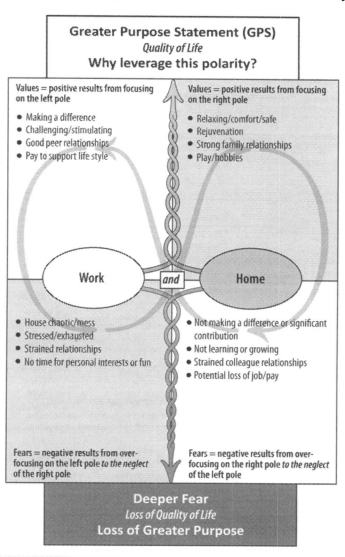

I have used this same Work and Home polarity exercise with thousands of colleagues in healthcare over the years, and the values and fears turn out to be fairly consistent:

- The upsides of Work: making a difference; having challenging/stimulating good relationships with people at work; and earning income to support one's lifestyle.
- The upsides of Home: having a relaxing/comfortable/safe place; taking time to rejuvenate; having strong family relationships; and enjoying leisure, play, and hobbies.

You can see on the completed map above that the downside of one pole is the loss of the upsides of the other pole. However, what matters most is *what you value* and *what you fear.*

NOTE: The infinity loop of a well-leveraged polarity has a large presence in the upper quadrants and small presence in the lower quadrants. The illustration above represents a well-leveraged polarity, because the infinity loop is sitting in upper quadrants and showing that there is support for maximizing the upsides and minimizing the downsides.

Reflection on the Work and Home Polarity

Have you ever focused on work to the neglect of your home life? What happened? Did the people you share your home with bring this to your attention? Have you ever come home from work and found a mess or a virtually empty refrigerator when everyone is hungry? Have you ever been at a family event and were so tired you could not enjoy it or had no energy for those activities you usually enjoy? Most of us know the downside of focusing on Work to the neglect of Home—all the things we love about Home seem to have disappeared. Notice what the infinity loop looks like when this is your reality:

The Infinity Loop: The Consequences of Favoring Work Over Home

Overemphasis on Work

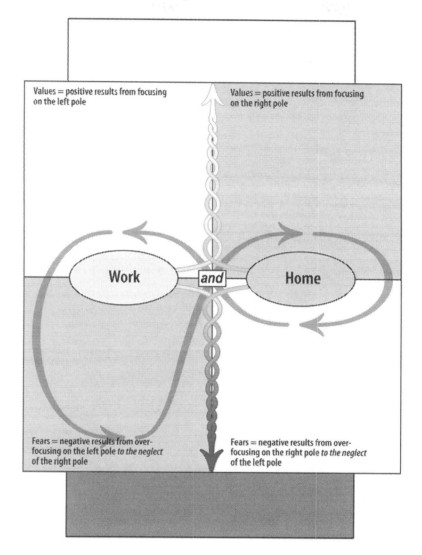

The concentration of tension moves into the downside quadrant of Work and is not moving to the Home pole *because you have neglected it*. It is often the fear of losing the valued positive outcomes of your preferred pole that explains why the other pole is essentially being ignored.

Now let us reverse the example. **Have you ever worked with someone who focuses on Home instead of Work?** What happened? Did their colleagues and teammates become frustrated or resentful because they had to take up the slack, leading to job stress and frayed relationships? When the focus is on Home, their job performance and initiative are likely to be dropping to the point where their jobs are in jeopardy. All the things they value about Work will be lost because they are not focusing on Work in equal measure as Home, as can be seen in the following illustration.

The Infinity Loop: The Consequences of Focusing Too Much on Home and Neglecting Work

Overemphasis on Home

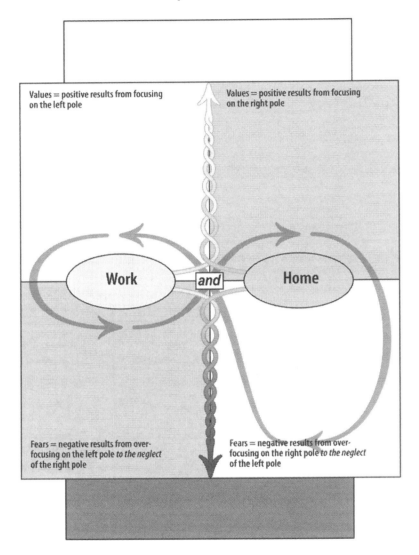

The results are always the same over time if you focus on one pole to the neglect of the other: **You will lose some or all of what you value in the other pole (obviously, this is the downside).** It becomes clear with this polarity that there is no one thing you can do to end the tension that exists between these poles because it is not a problem to be solved. It is instead a polarity that must be leveraged by focusing on each pole equally.

Ahead in Chapter 3:

Before we move deeper into the process of leveraging polarities, it would be good to look at one of our strongest and best skills as healthcare practitioners: **solving problems.**

Chapter 3

Traditional "Either/Or" Thinking Alone Puts Leaders at Risk

The leader noted that the concept of "both/and" is not only new but questionable. "What if I don't like the other pole? I have found that one of my accountabilities as a leader is to get everyone to be on the same page. It takes expertise to get others to think like you on some of the hard issues we deal with. I feel like this is one of my strengths. I think you are suggesting that 'both/and' is important. I get the feeling you are suggesting that I should be reaching out and encouraging others to stay strong in their pole. I'm not sure that will work."

The best healthcare practitioners and leaders are master problem solvers. We learned to solve problems as a way of demonstrating competency throughout our formal education. We learned how to spell words and how to add and subtract numbers, the names of important people in history, and the dates of important events. We learned about gravity in General Science and why things work the way they do. What we learn in the testing (problem-solving) process in formal education is that it is important to find the right or best answer as soon as possible. Those who solve problems quickly and correctly get high grades and high scores.

We learned two important lessons from all the problem-solving tests we were given in formal education:

1. When you are right, you get rewarded.

2. When you are right, those who disagree with you are wrong.

Lesson 1: Society rewards good problem solvers. They get "A" grades and often go on to college and graduate school. Within the healthcare community, the ability to make the right diagnosis and carry out the right treatment (solve problems) is critical. *Either* the symptoms lead us to one diagnosis, *or* they lead us to another. *Either* the swollen ankle that was twisted while running is sprained, *or* there is a more accurate diagnosis.

Solving the diagnosis problem will be used to shape the treatment program. Thousands of lives are saved every day through problem solving and either/or thinking. It is no wonder that healthcare workers are such good problem solvers and so skilled at either/or thinking. We can and should take great pride in that.

Lesson 2: The more convinced you are that you have the right answer, the more convinced you are that those who disagree with you are wrong. This natural assumption is a byproduct of the testing process in formal education. If 4 plus 4 equals 8, all other answers are wrong, right?

In healthcare, the more convinced I am that the collective symptoms lead to diagnosis A, the more convinced I am that diagnosis B, with a completely different set of symptoms, is wrong. Solving the problem of *either* diagnosis A *or* some other diagnosis, B *or* C *or* D, is essential. The ability to differentiate between options and select the right one or best one is the foundation of *either/or* problem solving. And, when your diagnosis is correct, it is logical that conflicting diagnoses are wrong. Knowing this frees us to move ahead with the correct treatment that includes some additional problems to solve involving *either/or* thinking. Now we are looking for the best combination of interventions, and we are again moving into choices of *either* this combination *or* some alternative combination.

Solving thousands of problems throughout our formal education helps us be good *either/or* problem solvers, and when we get into the clinical setting, those skills are strengthened even more. Thus, we have a set of skills based on years of formal education and years of practice. Yet these very skills—the ability to solve a range of problems *and* the ability to handle *either/or* dilemmas—are not enough by themselves to address the many situations in healthcare that require *both/and* thinking.

Many endemic problems can be broken down into sets of polarities that will require us to switch from *either/or* thinking to **both/and thinking.** When we rely on *either/or* problem solving to address the polarities in the rapidly changing work and life cultures of today, we will get what we always got. Is that what you want? We must do better.

The major issues haunting healthcare practitioners and institutions today are actually combinations of problems to be solved and values that are strengthened when they are managed together. This requires *both/and* thinking. We do not have the same track record for *both/and* thinking! It is harder for *either/or* thinkers to supplement it with *both/and* thinking because it is moving outside a model or framework that is deeply rooted in their success.

However, haven't we all been presented with alternatives that create tension? Sometimes we feel like we are caught between a rock and a hard place—either choice will get us in trouble. That is obviously a *dilemma.* Sometimes we hear a statement that seems to contradict itself, such as "The more things change, the more they stay the same," or "Less is more." The tension in the paradox often shows up when we feel like we have to choose. Life is full of tension-creating choices.

Polarities show up or are experienced as natural tensions between interdependent, competing, or different values that are unavoidable, unsolvable, and indestructible. They will always exist within the human condition; they are never going away. That's why we have to learn how to leverage them—not "fix" or "solve" them.

The Clinical Practice Model Resource Center created an International Consortium of colleagues committed to transform healthcare. The center brings colleagues from the consortium together to share the many lessons learned in their transformation work. In one of the learning sessions, 49 colleagues from 49 member institutions identified the 34 areas of attention and priority that should be managed as interdependent pairs of polarities. Here is their list of priorities needing immediate attention:

> The CPMRC Consortium identified these interdependent polarity pairs as priority values that should be managed with Polarity Thinking at the point of care:
>
> - Cost of Care (Margin) *and* Quality of Care (Mission)
> - Project-Driven Change *and* Framework-Driven Change
> - Staff Workloads *and* Patient Needs
> - Patient Safety *and* Staff Safety
> - Patient Satisfaction *and* Staff Satisfaction
> - Standardized Care *and* Autonomous Care
> - Medical Care *and* Whole-Person Care
> - Change *and* Stability
> - Conditional Respect *and* Unconditional Respect
> - Technology Platform *and* Practice Platform
> - Candor *and* Diplomacy
> - Individual Competency *and* Team Competency
> - Routine Task Accountability *and* Scope of Practice Accountability
> - Vertical/Hierarchical Relationships *and* Horizontal/Partnership Relationships
> - Directive Decision Making *and* Shared Decision Making
> - Retention of Staff *and* Recruitment of Staff
> - Physician Expectation *and* Administration Expectations

Each of the areas in the list above act as pole preferences that will create tension. If you use *either/or* thinking or treat one pole as the solution to a problem, you will get only a quick fix; the problem will eventually recur. This lack of success will lead to frustration, guilt, and possibly even blaming. Whether you blame yourself or you blame others, you are acting on the assumption that the problem is solvable and that failing to come up with a permanent solution is indicative of lack of will or intelligence. When the problem is part of an underlying polarity, you need to stop being hard on one another and take another approach.

The dominant thinking and comfort level in healthcare is with problems and quick fixes. We all feel better when we can find a quick solution to a problem—especially if it looks like a problem we settled before. But who becomes accountable if the fix doesn't work? And how much of your precious resources will be wasted before someone says *enough*? The accountability to leverage or manage polarities that never go away is a whole new pattern of thinking. It is a new logic; it is the missing link. It is hard to believe that one has been successful if a concern/issue never goes away. We all desire to have things "taken care of" or "moved off our plates."

One of the major differences between solving a problem the old way and using a relatively new approach like Polarity Thinking is that you have to be vigilant in the way you manage each polarity. Both poles have equal importance and need equal and continuous focus to strengthen each value so that you create the conditions under which the two can work together. Leveraging the polarities stops the ups and downs and the pendulum effects of initiatives that increase the chaos and stress in healthcare. Manage by leveraging and you will reach your desired outcomes and shared goals.

Polarity Thinking gives us back our optimism that we can stabilize and sustain those things that matter the most while the institution is making the necessary changes. Leveraging polarities shows us how to capitalize on these inherent tensions in healthcare facilities so that opposites reinforce each other, rather than fight each other. The polarity values stop being sources of chronic frustration and become models of excellence.

Problem-Solving Patterns

Because of our problem-solving background, we often think that what we need to do is convince others to agree with our point of view. We typically think that if we are very clear in communicating our perspective, others will support it. That worked well for *either/or* thinking, but not now. With polarities, the clearer you communicate your point of view (problem, solution, and strategy), *the greater the resistance will be from those holding the alternative point of view.* The downside of the pole you favor is not noticed by you, but it is especially noticed by others who prefer the other pole.

It is important to know which pole you prefer, because the strength of that affinity parallels with the fears you might have about the other pole's downside, which of course is the loss of the positive outcomes of your preference pole. *If your preference pole is very popular, it is most important to seek out and listen to the voices of those who prefer the other pole.* This will become clearer when we take a close look at diverse polarities and learn to leverage them.

Since each pole is very important, it is hard to spontaneously accept that all the hard work, concern, ideas, and resources being used to focus on one pole can actually make things worse *over time*. But that is exactly what will happen. This is an important paradox, and it is 100 percent predictable. Just pausing to reflect on what we know about problem solving helps us to remember to be vigilant when we are dealing with a polarity.

Make your tacit wisdom explicit, and then share it. I am not suggesting that that you have not been leveraging polarities all along or that you should run back to work and look for polarities to experiment with. On the contrary! You have been leveraging polarities all your life—in your families, in relationships with friends and loved ones, in your formal and informal education, and in your work as a healthcare professional. Remember when you were, oh, three or four years old and you played with your friends and your toys on the floor in the living room? All kids argue with other children from time to time over who is going to play with a certain toy. This time, it's your toy, and you want it. At this point, your mother or father steps in and tells you to do *what* with your toys? "SHARE!" I doubt that you were told that sharing is a polarity to leverage, but it is!

In all our lives, we go back to that early lesson: *How do I take care of my own wants and needs AND take care of the wants and needs of the people who are important to me?*

If I just take care of myself, I will be seen as selfish and will lose my friend, but if I just take care of my friend, I will feel neglected and resentful, and decide that my friend is selfish.

If we can look at the situation as a challenge to achieve win-win, we reach our greater purpose: a thriving relationship.

This example can be scaled up to a parallel organizational polarity in which we must do two things: Take care of our practice (Self) and take care of the patient (Other).

As in most situations involving competing values, we exacerbate the problem when we assume that we have to choose one or the other.

Polarities, dilemmas, paradoxes: they are so central to life that we work our way through them on a daily basis without realizing it. Most are simple and basic. It is this life experience and tacit wisdom you have acquired from leveraging these daily tensions that will help you understand and apply Polarity Thinking to more complex and endemic problems. You will have a user-friendly model and set of principles that can be applied to all polarities. Having a common model and set of principles makes it easier to work intentionally with others to tap the huge potential available when polarities are leveraged well.

Chapter 4

How to Leverage Polarities

"If you are asking the right questions, you are probably living the right answers."

— Rumi

The first question to ask when you become aware of a problematic situation at work is this: Is this a problem to be solved, or is this a polarity that needs to be leveraged? Or both? Remember that a problem and a polarity are not the same thing. *Is the situation an ongoing one, such as patient safety and staff safety?* (If so, it is a polarity.) *Does it have an end point?* Then it is not a polarity.

How to determine whether it is a problem or a polarity:

- Problems have an end point; polarities do not have an end point.

- Problems are not ongoing; polarities are ongoing.

- Problems are solvable; polarities are not solvable, they must be managed together.

- Problems have independent alternatives; polarities have *inter*dependent alternatives.

- Problems can stand alone; polarities cannot stand alone.

- With problems, there is no need to include an alternative for the solution to work. With polarities, the alternatives need one another to optimize the situation over time.

- Problems often contain mutually exclusive opposites, such as

  — Should we promote Chris? Yes or No
  — Should we remove one level of management? Yes or No

  Polarities always contain mutually *in*clusive opposites (i.e., Work and Home; Tough Love and Gentle Love; Competing and Collaborating; Mission and Margin).

Once a polarity is identified, you must do two things in order to successfully leverage it:

1. Take actions to make sure that each pole is strengthened (proactive).

2. Take action to make sure that you are not focusing too much on one pole to the neglect of the other (responsive).

We can no longer use the metaphor of Inhale and Exhale when talking about underlying principles related to leveraging polarities. Why? An intrinsic polarity like Inhale and Exhale is done automatically as long as the body system exists. Polarities, being unstoppable, infer that the tension will flow automatically. How much pain or joy will be generated in the process? How virtuous or vicious will the tension become? The oscillation between Inhale and Exhale is done *automatically* in the body. In all other polarities, it is essential to specifically take action steps to make sure that the positive values of each pole are supported. You must be vigilant and make sure that the tension movement will be *virtuous* rather than *vicious* by maximizing the upsides and minimizing the downsides.

Therefore, we now expand the map to include a vertical column placed alongside each pole. The column is divided into two parts: action steps and early warnings, as seen in the illustration that follows. This completes the polarity map.

A Complete Polarity Map

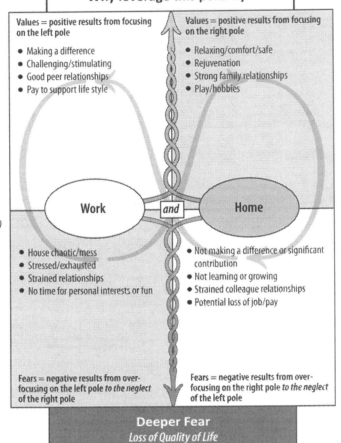

Action Steps
How will we gain or maintain the positive results from focusing on this left pole? What? Who? By when? Measures?

A. First Action Step

B. Second Action Step

Action Steps
How will we gain or maintain the positive results from focusing on this right pole? What? Who? By when? Measures?

A. First Action Step

B. Second Action Step

Early Warnings
Measurable indicators (things you can count) that will let you know that you are getting into the downside of this left pole.

A. First Early Warning

B. Second Early Warning

Early Warnings
Measurable indicators (things you can count) that will let you know that you are getting into the downside of this right pole.

A. First Early Warning

B. Second Early Warning

Greater Purpose Statement (GPS)
Quality of Life
Why leverage this polarity?

Values = positive results from focusing on the left pole

- Making a difference
- Challenging/stimulating
- Good peer relationships
- Pay to support life style

Values = positive results from focusing on the right pole

- Relaxing/comfort/safe
- Rejuvenation
- Strong family relationships
- Play/hobbies

Work *and* **Home**

- House chaotic/mess
- Stressed/exhausted
- Strained relationships
- No time for personal interests or fun

- Not making a difference or significant contribution
- Not learning or growing
- Strained colleague relationships
- Potential loss of job/pay

Fears = negative results from over-focusing on the left pole *to the neglect of the right pole*

Fears = negative results from over-focusing on the right pole *to the neglect of the left pole*

Deeper Fear
Loss of Quality of Life
Loss of Greater Purpose

Components of a complete polarity map:

- Eleven components of the Basic Map

- Action steps: steps that must be taken in order to strengthen or support each value (pole) simultaneously

- Early warnings: the symptoms when one pole is being neglected

Two Additional Components:
Action Steps and Early Warnings

Action Steps

The action steps are the interventions necessary to gain or maintain the desired positive outcomes of each pole and keep the tension/energy between the poles oscillating between the upper quadrants. This creates a virtuous movement to reach the greater purpose. It is a form of appreciative inquiry related to what is working or what is desired.

Action steps are listed on the map so that your point of view is known and supported. Sometimes it is easier to list what is needed to sustain or grow *your* preferred pole than it is to list the interventions needed to support the opposite pole. However, when the action steps are taken to support both poles, the result is a virtuous spiral to the greater purpose (which in this case is a fulfilling quality of life). **With this polarity, the action steps and early warnings need to be meaningful for you**. *You need to write your own.*

Early Warnings

Identifying the early warnings is a critical step in leveraging polarities. These signs are an early alert and are often measurable, so they help us recognize that the tension/energy flow between the poles is not being leveraged because the other pole is being neglected. **It is a warning that action is needed to prevent the tension/energy flow from going in the wrong direction**—to the downside—resulting in the negative outcomes or fears that are visible on the map.

Early warnings are visible and measurable. They let you know that you are getting into the downsides of a pole. Paying attention to the early warnings on each pole prevents us from going into the vicious downward spiral leading to the deeper fear/concern (which in this case is decreased quality of life).

We return to the Work and Home example introduced earlier in the chapter and provide a completed map for the additional components of action steps and early warnings.

Completed Map for Work and Home Polarity with Action Steps and Early Warnings

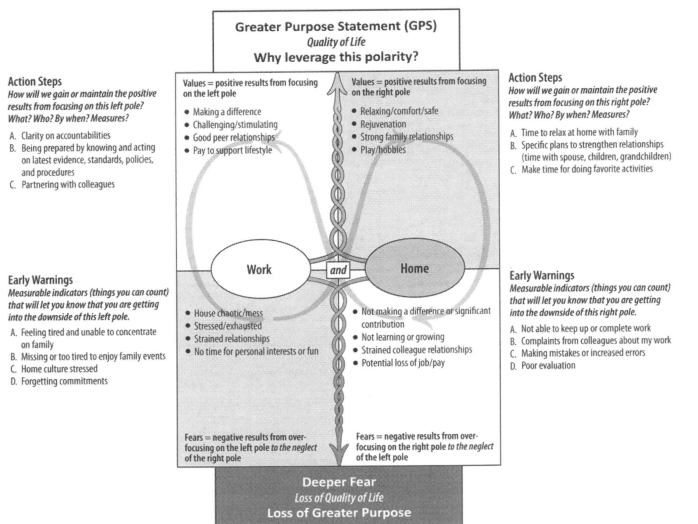

Greater Purpose Statement (GPS)
Quality of Life
Why leverage this polarity?

Action Steps
How will we gain or maintain the positive results from focusing on this left pole? What? Who? By when? Measures?

A. Clarity on accountabilities
B. Being prepared by knowing and acting on latest evidence, standards, policies, and procedures
C. Partnering with colleagues

Action Steps
How will we gain or maintain the positive results from focusing on this right pole? What? Who? By when? Measures?

A. Time to relax at home with family
B. Specific plans to strengthen relationships (time with spouse, children, grandchildren)
C. Make time for doing favorite activities

Values = positive results from focusing on the left pole

- Making a difference
- Challenging/stimulating
- Good peer relationships
- Pay to support lifestyle

Values = positive results from focusing on the right pole

- Relaxing/comfort/safe
- Rejuvenation
- Strong family relationships
- Play/hobbies

Work *and* **Home**

Early Warnings
Measurable indicators (things you can count) that will let you know that you are getting into the downside of this left pole.

A. Feeling tired and unable to concentrate on family
B. Missing or too tired to enjoy family events
C. Home culture stressed
D. Forgetting commitments

- House chaotic/mess
- Stressed/exhausted
- Strained relationships
- No time for personal interests or fun

- Not making a difference or significant contribution
- Not learning or growing
- Strained colleague relationships
- Potential loss of job/pay

Early Warnings
Measurable indicators (things you can count) that will let you know that you are getting into the downside of this right pole.

A. Not able to keep up or complete work
B. Complaints from colleagues about my work
C. Making mistakes or increased errors
D. Poor evaluation

Fears = negative results from over-focusing on the left pole *to the neglect of the right pole*

Fears = negative results from over-focusing on the right pole *to the neglect of the left pole*

Deeper Fear
Loss of Quality of Life
Loss of Greater Purpose

Ask yourself these two questions about leveraging polarities:

1. What action steps do we need to take to proactively gain the benefits of each pole? When each pole is supported, you are leveraging the tension necessary to reach the greater purpose.

2. What are the early warnings that help us see that one pole is getting all the attention, to the neglect of the other pole? Pay attention to the early warnings in order to prevent falling to the deeper fear.

Action Steps: Look over the completed map shown above. The action steps here are intended to keep the Work pole strong: clarify your work accountabilities; prepare by knowing and acting on latest evidence, standards, policies, and procedures; and partner with colleagues. For the Home pole, write down specific times to relax at home, strengthen relationships, and make time for favorite activities.

Early Warnings: Let's assume the preference pole is Work, the left pole. No one would deny that work has many positive outcomes. The first people to notice that you are focusing on work and neglecting your home life will be your spouse, someone in your family, or a friend. If you need help, they will be the ones to help you list the early warnings that show you are over-focusing on work.

Some examples of early warnings that you are focusing on work at the neglect of home are: You and others will notice you are feeling tired and unable to concentrate on family, you are missing or too tired to enjoy family events, and the stress from the work environment is making you forget home commitments. The early warnings are often comments being made from those who are a part of the culture around you because they are usually the first to experience the downside of your dominant pole.

However, you would be the one who could list the early warnings that there is too much focus on home, resulting in work being neglected, such as, you are not able to keep up or complete your work, colleagues are complaining about your work, you are making mistakes or increased errors and receiving poor evaluations.

Quick Fixes vs. Solutions Sustained "Over Time"

Finding solutions that are still working over a sustained period of time is an important goal in Polarity Thinking. The early warnings keep us from slipping back into our problem-solving mode of thinking and remind us that *either/or* will not work for polarities. As we all know, healthcare professionals love quick fixes—they are embedded in our culture. The quick-fix mindset is especially evident just before a certification review team arrives or the Public Health Department has to do an inspection. Everyone is running around fixing things so that everything looks good and meets the standards. Implementing a new mandatory form before the reviewers arrive is a popular quick fix, but two months later, someone notices that the new form is not being used anymore. Apparently it worked for a while, but was abandoned because it did not fix the underlying problems.

There are no quick fixes with polarities. That is a hard reality to accept, because we are so used to fixing things! If the staff had first acknowledged that the situation is not really a problem to be solved but instead a matter of getting two competing values in sync with action steps and early warnings, success would be achieved. Had they balanced the two values by focusing on the pole that is being neglected and assessed whether or not the short-term and long-term strategies listed under the action steps are being carried out or are inadequate, they would achieve success.

In the *either/or* mindset, when things don't work, we know right away that the choice was not good and that we will come up with one that fixes the problem. The early warnings are constant reminders that you want solutions that work over time, and that means that both poles need to be managed simultaneously or you will experience the downside of the very pole you saw as the fix. Early warnings remind us of this.

Polarity Thinking is about reaching and *sustaining* a greater purpose. Sustaining requires an ongoing form of self-correction guided by the early warnings. If one pole is seen as a problem to solve or fix and there is no self-correction to the other pole, you will have a so-called fix, but a fix that is a failure. Most of us have experienced implementing a good idea that worked for a while but over time proved not to be so good. It is a symptom that the real issue is a polarity not a problem.

Interdependence is an over-time concept. It may seem foreign to think of very different or alternatives or opposites as connected or interdependent. That is why the pendulum effect is familiar in healthcare. It comes in the form of new initiatives. The pendulum is associated with extremes that we never thought of as interdependent *over time*. The pendulum is associated with movement from one side to the other. It is hard to believe that "over time" a good idea has limitations, yet we see it often. We watch programs come and go, and what seemed good for a while did not last. We focus on one pole as a problem to solve, and when that fails, we focus on the other side as a problem, all of which wastes time, money, and resources. *The downsides can be avoided.*

The Work and Home polarity will never go away as long as you are working, and quality of life affects all areas of our lives on a daily basis and over the long term. All interdependent pairs can be managed the same way the Work and Home pair in this chapter can be managed. The fundamentals are the same. Once you have a basic understanding of Polarity Thinking and how to use the map, you can use the approach with all polarities, personal and professional, to address chronic problems and dilemmas that surround us every day.

The polarity map and all its components are generically explained. The next few chapters will extend our discussion of polarities by focusing on some common examples to deepen understanding of how to use the Polarity Thinking approach.

Explanation of Polarity Map Components

Greater Purpose Statement (GPS)
*The virtuous cycle creates the behavior/outcomes
that neither pole can do alone*
Why leverage this polarity?

Action Steps
How will we gain or maintain the positive results from focusing on this left pole? What? Who? By when? Measures?

A. Action steps are the interventions necessary to maintain and sustain the desired positive behaviors/outcomes of each pole.
B. Action steps keep the tension/energy between the poles oscillating within the upper quadrants.

Action Steps
How will we gain or maintain the positive results from focusing on this right pole? What? Who? By when? Measures?

A. Action steps leverage the energy and prevent the flow from going to the downside.
B. Action steps minimize the downside outcomes.
C. Action steps prevent the pendulum effect.

Values = positive results from focusing on the left pole
- Reflects the value or desired behaviors/outcomes associated with this pole and is called the UPSIDE.
- Desired behaviors/outcomes will only appear if the Action Steps necessary to achieve these outcomes are acted on.

Values = positive results from focusing on the right pole
- Reflects the value or desired behaviors/outcomes associated with this pole and is called the UPSIDE.
- The tension and energy flow is driven by experiencing or anticipating the downside of one pole combined with the attraction to the upside of the other pole.

Neutral Pole *and* **Neutral Pole**

Early Warnings
Measurable indicators (things you can count) that will let you know that you are getting into the downside of this left pole.

A. Warning signs are an alert that the energy/tension between the poles is not being leveraged because the other pole is being neglected.
B. Often, the warning signs are comments made by those who are part of the culture around you because they are often the first to experience the downside of your dominant role.

Early Warnings
Measurable indicators (things you can count) that will let you know that you are getting into the downside of this right pole.

A. It is a warning that action is needed in order to prevent the energy flow to the downside resulting in the negative behaviors/outcomes or fears that are visible.
B. Signs to help us prevent slipping back into our problem-solving modes of thinking and remind us that either/or will not work for polarities.

- Reflects the negative behaviors/outcomes associated with the loss of the positive outcomes of the Right pole.
- Makes transparent the legitimate fears or loss of the positive outcomes of the Right pole.

- Reflects the negative behaviors/outcomes associated with the loss of the positive behaviors/outcomes of the Left pole.
- Makes transparent the legitimate fears or loss of the positive outcomes of the Left pole.

Fears = negative results from over-focusing on the left pole *to the neglect of the right pole*

Fears = negative results from over-focusing on the right pole *to the neglect of the left pole*

Deeper Fear
Neglect of either pole creates the vicious cycle leading to the opposite of the GPS
Loss of Greater Purpose

Chapter 5

Leveraging Patient Satisfaction and Staff Satisfaction

A director in a large Midwest healthcare system was describing an "aha" moment. He recalled a meeting he attended and said, "One of the items on the agenda was patient satisfaction. What immediately passed in front of me was a meeting held 30 years ago in another state, and the main focus of that meeting was patient satisfaction. I remember thinking, Will this issue ever go away? I didn't know the answer was NO, it will never go away. I didn't know it was not a problem to solve, but a pole of a polarity that needed to be leveraged."

Every *successful* organization makes patient/customer/client satisfaction part of its mission statement. However, most think of this area as a "problem," which is why hundreds of millions of dollars are spent each year on customer satisfaction programs and initiatives. The ways organizations and institutions go about improving or fixing their customer relationships are remarkably similar all across the country. For example, the CEO or leadership team issues a mandate, and the entire organization focuses on the initiative. Whether the board of directors pressures the leadership team to increase market share or the company feels pressured to strengthen its regional reputation for quality care, these programs are high-profile efforts.

When it comes to patient satisfaction, we see patterns of behavior that look like this:

- The middle managers are given the directives and told that they will be held accountable for the success or failure of the effort.

- They are told to report their progress at monthly meetings to review the status and outcomes of this priority strategic goal.

- Evaluations and bonuses are connected to the effort.

- The middle managers give the results of the patient satisfaction scores to the staff, and each department's numbers are compared to other units within the system.

- Awards and recognition are given to those staff members or teams who are showing improvement or presenting the highest scores.

The outcomes? Variable. In this chapter, we present a clinical case study and use a polarity map to clarify the systemic ramifications of "misdiagnosing" a polarity for a problem.

A Clinical Scenario:

The CEO was irritated: "How is it that I have spent 1.7 million dollars on our strategic goal to increase customer satisfaction and ended up in this mess?" The story began when the board discussed with him that the patient satisfaction was unacceptable and they were going to be losing their market share if something wasn't done about it. They expected him to address this immediately.

I asked him what he said when he left the boardroom. He replied that he assured them that he would "fix this problem." "What did you do?" I asked. He explained that he called a special mandatory meeting for the entire leadership team—a large group consisting of VPs, directors, and managers—and told them that he expected them to come back in a week with new ideas and ways they intended to increase patient satisfaction. He let them know that he was going to go around the room, every person will present their ideas, and they will discuss approaches.

The next week, everyone arrived with a plan. One individual mentioned that he knew of a customer satisfaction program they could purchase that was showing good outcomes. They decided to purchase the program.

The action steps within the satisfaction program were to put every staff through an all-day workshop, focusing on suggestions as to what to say and how to work differently with the patients and family. The CEO described the results:

> The staff didn't even appreciate the in-services! We gave rewards and recognition for the climbing patient satisfaction. We followed the program guidelines. We did everything right, and now it is 18 months later and the patient satisfaction is lower than it was before we began the program! And the staff morale has been steadily declining. What's wrong with this picture? What's wrong with these people?

What went wrong?

It started back in the boardroom when he promised them he would "fix this problem" and support the goal to be the provider of choice (another name for the outcomes of customer/client/patient satisfaction pole). Since he saw it as a problem to solve, he brought together his whole team to help him fix it. Everyone agreed that patient/client satisfaction is an important priority. There was also an understanding by the managers that if they did not improve customer satisfaction, it could put the system in financial stress. ***No one knew this was a polarity to be managed.***

The clinical scenario just described becomes the basis for our next look at managing polarities.

The completed map on the following page shows the upsides of the Patient/Client Satisfaction pole (left upper quadrant): patients and families feel that their individual needs are being met and that they, the patients, are considered to be an important part of their care. When the patients feel this way, they will talk to their neighbors and friends in the community about how well they were treated.

Completed Map for the Patient/Client Satisfaction and Staff Satisfaction Polarity

Greater Purpose Statement (GPS)
Best place to give and receive care
Why leverage this polarity?

Action Steps
How will we gain or maintain the positive results from focusing on this left pole? What? Who? By when? Measures?

A. Orientation, performance expectation reinforces the importance of patient's story, partnership with patient and family, and integrated team
B. Mutuality and review of plan of care at the beginning of each shift
C. Staff review feedback from patient's satisfaction surveys and integrate into practice improvements
D. Engage patient/family in the coordination of their individualized care

Values = positive results from focusing on the left pole

- Patient care/service is individualized and integrated across team.
- Patient families are engaged with staff in the planning and delivery of care that brings excellent outcomes.
- Patients talk highly of care/service received.

Values = positive results from focusing on the right pole

- Staff feel valued and recognized for their contributions and expertise.
- Staff are engaged in decision making that enhances their ability to deliver quality care/service.
- The organization provides resources for ongoing staff development.
- The hospital is considered an excellent place to work.

Action Steps
How will we gain or maintain the positive results from focusing on this right pole? What? Who? By when? Measures?

A. Strong partnership infrastructure.
B. Engage in decision making that improves the environment and care processes.
C. Tools, resources, and infrastructures to support evidence-based interdisciplinary, integrated care are supporting staff in work processes.
D. Provide continuous learning opportunities.
E. A process exists to provide recognition and positive feedback for performance.

Patient/Client Satisfaction *and* **Staff Satisfaction**

Early Warnings
Measurable indicators (things you can count) that will let you know that you are getting into the downside of this left pole.

A. "What do they think we are doing here, running a hotel?"
B. "If we don't have what we need to give quality care, we can't meet patients' needs."
C. "What we think doesn't matter around here, only what patients think."
D. "We aren't supported to attend needed ongoing education and skill building sessions."

- Staff do not feel valued or recognized for their contributions and expertise.
- Staff feel decisions around important practice issues and work environments are made without their input.
- Resources for staff development are limited.
- Staff do not feel it is a good place to work.

- Care/service is becoming less focused on patients' individualized needs.
- Staff decide what is best for patients and families without their input.
- Decrease in patient satisfaction (i.e., increase in complaints, poor outcomes of care, increased length of stay).

Early Warnings
Measurable indicators (things you can count) that will let you know that you are getting into the downside of this right pole.

A. "I feel like a room number or a disease."
B. "My family and I do not feel listened to."
C. "Patient satisfaction scores are dropping."
D. Clinical indicators and scorecard results are changing in an unwanted way.

Fears = negative results from over-focusing on the left pole *to the neglect of the right pole*

Fears = negative results from over-focusing on the right pole *to the neglect of the left pole*

Deeper Fear
Not a good place to give or receive care
Loss of Greater Purpose

The map also shows the loss of this pole: Care and services are being delivered based only on *the staff's concerns,* rather than the concerns of the patient and his or her family. The staff is not engaging them in decisions and is not getting patient input, resulting in patients who do not feel that they are being cared about, and this is a big part of patient dissatisfaction.

The organization's preferred pole here is Patient Satisfaction, accompanied by a strong fear of the loss of the preference values (the downside of the Staff Satisfaction pole). The staff members were not familiar with polarities, so no one was asked this important question: "Is this a polarity, a problem, or both?" The staff saw Patient Satisfaction as a problem to solve and the only thing that needed their attention, so they were not also focusing of Staff Satisfaction.

Lessons Learned

When all the effort is focused on one pole, the inevitable will happen: It will generate its own resistance. There is less chance of attaining the goal, and even if by chance the goal is met, it will take more time and probably more resources than necessary, and the fix will be unsustainable *over time.*

Action Steps for the Patient Satisfaction Pole

The outcomes in this real-world scenario were 100% predictable, and the polarity map explains the outcomes. The team had clear action steps for the Patient Satisfaction pole.

- Staff members were assigned to mandatory in-service training that was focused on learning how to be more attentive to the patients and family.

- The education funds were targeted to support this work for every unit.

- The managers knew the importance of this goal and the organization's expectations (they too were being evaluated on their unit's improvement). Whenever the managers met with staff, patient satisfaction was on the top of the agenda.

- Emphasis was placed on training. People were questioned when they missed an education class. Signs, posters, reminders, and celebration notes were visible throughout the unit.

Early Warnings: Overemphasis on Patient Satisfaction

The CEO shared that initially the patient satisfaction scores improved, but slowly. Then gradually they plateaued. At the same time, he had another problem: staff dissatisfaction. People were making comments such as "What do you think we are running here, a hotel?" "We could give better care if we had the supplies and resources we need." "It doesn't matter what we think around here."

These early warnings *that the Patient Satisfaction pole was being focused on at the neglect of the Staff Satisfaction pole* were evident but since they did not know this was a polarity they kept pounding at the action steps to support patient satisfaction.

It is natural to resist any change effort that does not acknowledge the opposite pole, no matter how much sense it would make. Patient satisfaction is not bad, in fact it is very important, but it is simply not enough.

We can learn a lot about human resistance from looking at the natural tension that exists between interdependent pairs; this tension between poles can instill resistance. It makes sense that if one strongly values personal job satisfaction yet the organization is putting all its effort and attention around patient satisfaction and neglecting staff satisfaction, an employee might conclude that his or her efforts are not valued by the employer. If that is indeed the case, the employee is likely to resist any change effort focused only on patient satisfaction, despite understanding that it is important that the patients are satisfied. Understanding polarities changes everything.

Background of Our Scenario

Before the patient satisfaction program got off the ground, staff members were vocal about the hospital not doing enough to support their job satisfaction. No wonder patient satisfaction numbers were low before the program started! There is a clear correlation between staff satisfaction and customer satisfaction. If the staff members are not satisfied, the patients will not be satisfied. Therefore the more attention given to the Patient Satisfaction pole, the greater the resistance that came from the staff who were not feeling supported before the program was even initiated. The hospital did not respond to the staff adequately, and the resentment that was simmering before the program even started grew into staff resistance. Before long, the inevitable happened: they first experienced the downside of the Patient Satisfaction pole coupled with the downside of both poles as seen in the illustration on the following page.

Consequences of Over-Focusing on Patient Satisfaction and Neglecting to Focus Adequately on Staff Satisfaction

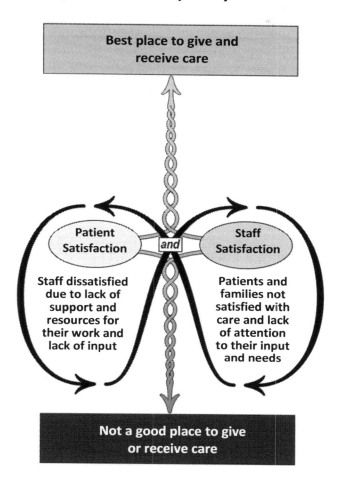

Resistance (early warnings) *is evidence that a strong value is being threatened.* Resistance will be present if a person is living in the downside of the very pole that is being focused on. The stronger the personal experience of living in the downside of a dominant pole, the greater the resistance will be to the action steps taken to support the pole. For example, if staff members feel any sense of neglect of their needs and notice that patient satisfaction gets a disproportionate amount of attention, they will not rally behind the action steps (resistance), despite the merit of the patient satisfaction program.

The resistance to the program is the result of the fear, the truths that the staff know about the downside of the Patient Satisfaction pole, the loss of their preference pole. However, the remedy is not to simply abandon the patient satisfaction action plan, but to supplement it with a staff satisfaction plan. If we do not *intentionally* pay attention to both poles at the same time, the negative consequences to the dominant pole will soon be followed by negative consequences to its counterpart pole. That is what happened in this situation.

Benefits and Consequences

Accurate diagnoses are at the core of any successful change. Again, the first step in accurate diagnosis is to be sure that the issue that needs attention is either a problem to be solved or a polarity that is not being managed well—or both. If a wrong diagnosis is made, there are definitive negative ramifications.

If you think a situation represents a problem to be solved but it really is a polarity, you will have the following nonintended consequences:

1. There will be resistance, which is going to impede progress.

2. Those who prefer one pole over the other will be protective about their preferred pole and feel those who resist it are wrong. This increases conflict and both might be more adamant about protecting their value.

3. Hierarchical power might be asserted to make a change happen (such as a mandate from the corporate office). Attainable and positive outcomes will not be sustained, and over time the negative outcomes will increase.

4. If the situation reveals a polarity but is being handled as a problem to be solved, it is worse than a waste of time. It is destructive, which means you pay twice.

Misdiagnosing the situation in any of the ways covered in this chapter can lead to power struggles between the two poles. First, in this power struggle, relationships can be harmed, jobs can be lost, and energy will almost surely be spent trying to win the power struggle. Second, even if one group indeed "wins," the system is positioned to eventually get the downsides of the winners' preferred pole. In the argument over inhaling and exhaling, it does not matter who wins: the organization will be blue in the face in a short time! Third, when winners are persistent in their attempts to hold on to their pole, eventually it will lead to the downside of both poles.

Leveraging the Tension

To prevent all these consequences, you must begin to leverage the tension between the poles. When polarities are managed well, the resistance turns into a determination to catapult to a greater purpose—something both poles value. In the case of this Patient/Staff Satisfaction polarity, the greater purpose is to "**Make the hospital the best place to give and receive care.**" There is a natural tension present in all polarities—in fact, it is what keeps life interesting. Natural tension is a part of life, so use it to facilitate life, not interfere with it. To effectively make the most of this natural tension, you must recognize how it manifests itself and use it to mobilize the people and the efforts that you know will create and strengthen the desired outcomes.

Polarity Thinking increases the speed of all change. When people see what they value being honored and supported, they are more likely to want to prevent the downside of the opposite pole, thus there is no more need to resist. Once the fears of the downside are identified, people become less fearful of change. Most importantly, the desired outcomes or the higher purpose can be sustained over time.

Positive Outcomes of an Accurate Diagnosis

When you know a situation represents polarities you can leverage, you immediately know many things:

- All the components in Polarity Thinking are applicable to your situation.

- Just knowing the way it works influences our behavior. It changes the power in relationships immediately, because we know that we must intentionally support both poles.

- It becomes easier to identify the other pole, ask questions to clarify the positives for each pole, and take actions to support both.

- Attainability of desired outcomes occurs more readily because resistance is decreased. The natural tension between the poles can be used to help achieve the greater purpose and ensure sustainability.

Knowing polarities exist gives us a sensitivity to recognize them early.

Chapter 6

Leveraging the Change and Stability Polarity

"Be the change you wish to see in the world."
— Gandhi

Once there is an understanding of polarities, it becomes apparent there are numerous polarities that relate to the individual and the internal phases and changes that we experience throughout our lives. We know they show up in various ways such as excitement and avoidance, complaints, conflicts, and resistance to change. Change is the only constant all humans can count on. Polarities are everywhere because change is everywhere.

Change is also a major constant for anyone associated with healthcare. The Institute of Medicine (IOM) report noted that the changes needed to create a sustainable healthcare system for this society are profound and the work is an urgent, achievable priority that needs resources. The report also noted that the reason most change has not been effective or sustainable is because it was not based on principles to guide it.

This chapter is so important because

1. few are aware that change is not a problem to be solved but a polarity that needs to be leveraged, and

2. few are aware of the principle of Polarity Thinking to guide their action steps.

Whenever change shows up, polarities are present. It is imperative that those who lead healthcare transformation understand the Change and Stability polarity. It is what I call a *mother polarity* because it is fundamental to all humanity. Mother polarities are personal and universal. They bear generic names. Here are a few such polarities: Change and Stability, Part and Whole, Self and Other, Local and Global, and Candor and Diplomacy.

We have come to know that each pole of a polarity calls for action steps that reflect the need for change at a personal and organizational level. The real challenge in health-care is that often the action steps call for change in behaviors by each member of the team who needs tools and resources to make that happen.

We will examine the importance of strengthening our ability to effect change and at the same time maintain internal and external stability within a system. The Change/Stability polarity is a very critical interdependent pair, particularly for those of us who are committed to making patients' lives and healthcare institutions better through healthcare transformation. The values of Change and Stability are values we all hold in common as human beings, but also as today's leaders in the industry. Like it or not, change and stability are not always things we can control professionally or personally, but the two can be managed and leveraged so that we reap the benefits of each equally. This polarity pair is the focus of this chapter.

Completed Map for Change and Stability Polarity

Greater Purpose Statement (GPS)

Why leverage this polarity?

Action Steps
How will we gain or maintain the positive results from focusing on this left pole? What? Who? By when? Measures?

A. Ensure that any changes being met are not violating the fundamental principles of the organization's mission and vision.
B. Explore how changes will positively support core tradition, beliefs, and organizational performance while advancing mission.
C. Avoid quick fixes and determine if the change is related to a problem to be solved or an effort to manage a polarity.
D. Evaluate the sustainability of the positive outcomes of the change.
E. Encourage innovation and creative thinking in all areas and provide resources to support this exploration.

Early Warnings
Measurable indicators (things you can count) that will let you know that you are getting into the downside of this left pole.

A. "I cannot keep up with the changes around here."
B. "We used to have more in common around our values and beliefs."
C. "Get on the train or we'll leave without you."
D. "Don't be bothered by the change; it will be gone and we'll be onto something else soon."
E. "All we do is change and things get more confusing and nothing improves. Who thinks up these ideas anyway?"
F. "There is so much going on around here we can't get our regular work done."

Values = positive results from focusing on the left pole
- The change efforts in the organization bring new energy, excitement, and hope for improvement.
- Our organization invites openness to new ideas leading to innovation.
- We are flexible and responsive to continuous learning and improving care/services.

Change

Frequent change is increasing the chaos and a feeling of being unsafe and overwhelmed.
- Change is weakening our traditional values related to quality of care.
- The declining support for traditional values and increasing foolish risks are decreasing our organizational pride.

Fears = negative results from over-focusing on the left pole *to the neglect* of the right pole

Values = positive results from focusing on the right pole
- Our traditional values are supported, giving us a sense of comfort, safety, and predictability.
- Our team is clear about the traditional values that sustain quality healthcare.
- We are proud of our organization's expertise based on past and present values, traditions, and wisdom.

and

Stability

- We are experiencing a stagnation and boredom in our culture.
- Our team is closed to new ideas, new thinking.
- Our loss of flexibility and responsiveness has resulted in missed opportunities for improvement, growth, and new learning.

Fears = negative results from over-focusing on the right pole *to the neglect* of the left pole

Action Steps
How will we gain or maintain the positive results from focusing on this right pole? What? Who? By when? Measures?

A. Provide opportunities to clarify what matters most to everyone on the team (core belief review).
B. Provide tools and resources to live the things that matter most in daily work life.
C. Performance reviews are based on individuals living what matters most.
D. Recognize those who live core values.

Early Warnings
Measurable indicators (things you can count) that will let you know that you are getting into the downside of this right pole.

A. "All we do is complain, but nothing gets done."
B. "We are stuck in the mud of how it has always been done around here."
C. "These change agents are getting in the way of doing our work here."

Deeper Fear

Loss of Greater Purpose

Reflections on the Change and Stability Polarity

Upsides. The upsides of the Change pole are familiar to all of us: there is energy and direction, creativity, excitement, and hope for improvement and growth. As for Stability, it honors things that matter most and gives us a sense of safety, predictability, and continuity when it comes to those traditions fundamental to our commitment to give our patients the very best care possible.

Change. The healthcare system as a whole is undergoing an intense period of change. Many healthcare professionals are living in the downside of the Change pole. It is not uncommon to hear colleagues bring forth the early warnings, showing there is an over-focus on the change pole. Here are typical comments when changes are introduced in a facility on a regular basis without a widespread understanding of the need for it or the rationale that prompted the specific changes.

People complain to one another. *"I can't keep up with the changes." "It seems like all we do is change. One day we do it this way, the next day a different way." "All we do is change and things get more confusing and nothing improves." "Who thinks up these ideas, anyway?" "What ever happened to the basics?" "We don't have a common ground on important things, and you never know what is going to happen next."*

Comments from staff members are the early warnings that alert us to something gone wrong. One of the poles is being neglected in favor of the other. The natural tension is not oscillating between the upper quadrants on the map. Instead, it is falling into the downside of Change, as seen in the figure below. The greater purpose, to have a flexible, strong, vibrant learning organization, cannot be reached.

Overemphasis on Change to the Neglect of Stability

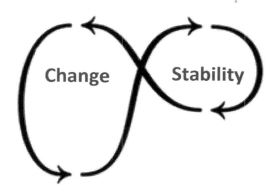

Ironically, most people who value Change do not realize that Stability is also part of their success. If you are someone who values and knows the importance of change and the energy, excitement, and hope for improvement that comes with it, you are no doubt very clear about the downside of stability (the pole on the right) and fear the "stagnation" that comes with it.

Change is integral to solving the many problems that get in the way of what we are committed to doing: providing quality care.

Stability

The people who prefer the Stability pole want clear values around things that matter most. They also want a sense of comfort and safety with the "known," and predictability and continuity of values. They are proud of their expertise and the traditions that are at the foundation of the organization.

Equally important are their fears of the downside of the Change pole. *Often when people share with you why they prefer one pole over another, they start out with what they know is the downside of the opposite pole.* Remember: one pole represents the values we prefer and the fear of loss of those values (the downside of the opposite pole). The resistance around Change is nothing more than the fear that if Change is focused on to the neglect of Stability, they will get caught in the downside of Change (living in chaos, loss of values and traditions that matter most, discomfort and concern for safety, living in the "unknown," loss of continuity, constant readjustment, and feeling overwhelmed, overworked, and uncertain about their expertise). **Therefore, they will resist the change, even if it is good change.**

It is easy to think of those who value Stability as "barriers" to successful Change. When such people resist Change, it is hard to see that their reaction is actually an early warning that needs attention. It is easier to see the resistance as a weakness in those who value Stability. Without understanding polarities, you cannot leverage the dynamic tension between the poles, and therefore cannot achieve the greater purpose. Action steps to support each pole are needed, as seen in the completed Change and Stability polarity map. The greater purpose needs to speak to *both* poles. Most of us want to work in a flexible, strong, vibrant learning organization, and those who favor one pole over the other in such cultures will work to achieve that common goal.

One of the greatest advantages to using a polarity map is that it makes the downside of each pole visible. *Walk your talk,* we are told, but why is that so hard for some people? The polarity map explains that reality: when there is strong preference for one pole, there is an equally strong aversion for the downside of the other pole, which is the loss of one's values. When it appears that the other pole is interfering with the preferred pole or their pole is not as strong as it should be, they will not support the interventions—the actions necessary to strengthen the other pole. They will stay vigilant to their pole.

We often make our promises from our deep values, but our actions are more a reflection of our fears. This is apparent in the real world, so it is helpful to remember that when you are afraid of the downside of a pole, you are not the first to be afraid. Nor are you the only one who fears the consequences if you mess things up—it is a normal phenomenon that comes with being human. Polarity Thinking makes that fear transparent and provides a formal process for taking action (action steps) to prevent those real downsides from happening.

The Importance of Closely Managing the Change and Stability Polarity

Jim Collins, author of *Built to Last,* gave us a powerful example of the importance of managing change and stability at the same time. He contrasted the difference between what he called "Silver" companies (those that outperformed the stock market by a factor of 2) and "Gold" companies (those that outperformed the stock market by a factor of 10). His conclusion was that the "Gold" companies were better able to leverage the polarity of "Preserve the Core *and* Stimulate Progress." Collins used those words 20 years ago, but the concept of managing the two in equal measure is just as important, though we shorten the polarity pair to Change and Stability. We can use different names for the poles, but we are talking about the same concept: "preserve the core" is one way to define Stability, and "stimulate progress" is one way to think about Change.

Rita Gunther McGrath, an organizational theorist and professor of management at Columbia Business School, analyzed a 10-year study of public companies with market capitalization greater than $1 billion and found similar results: only 10 companies in her review grew their bottom line by 5% every year over the 10-year period. The winning organizations were all very different from one another, but the common thread that united them was their ability to manage continuity and transformation. This underscores the importance of the Stability (Continuity) and Change (Transformation) polarity pair and explains why millions of dollars have been wasted on change efforts.

Most people who love the Change pole do not see the value of the Stability pole. Equally important is that they do not look for the polarities that are underlying the problems that they hope to address with change. If you see something as a problem to solve but it is really a polarity, it will NOT be sustainable over time, no matter how good the intention for the change is and no matter how much money and effort you put into the change.

Change should be designed to reach and sustain a greater purpose or a desired goal. There is a difference between attainability (where you reach some goals) and sustainability (where this achievement lasts over time).

The first step of any successful change effort is to determine whether it is change made in order to solve a problem, a change intended to help manage a polarity, or both. If one does not accurately diagnose the situation, it is more than likely that the change effort will fail over time.

In any change effort, Stability and Change are at play. Every change effort needs the stability dimension for sustainability over time.

Polarities are neutral and unsolvable because no one side in a polarity pair is more important than the other. Being able to leverage the best in each one decreases resistance to change and increases the ability to sustain the positive outcomes of change.

- Leveraging helps us quickly identify polar tensions within complex situations.
- Leveraging both poles strengthens our appreciation for the natural tension.
- Leveraging both poles reduces conflict between individuals and groups.

Seeing the change as part of a polarity increases attainability, speed, and sustainability. Treating a polarity as if it were a problem to solve reduces the attainability and slows down the process by increasing resistance, and even if the resistance is overcome, the goal of the change is inherently unsustainable over time.

I believe that the concepts that make up the foundation of Polarity Thinking are fundamental for successful change and that leaders in healthcare management must be able to apply the techniques to meet their institutional goals. Change is a constant, but we are living in a time when the pressure to make fundamental changes far exceeds our need to cling to or rely on traditional ways of thinking. We need to take more time to assess apparent "problems" and involve our colleagues and staff members in the search for solutions that are effective over the long term. New initiatives and new projects need to be carefully balanced and managed so as to also preserve and strengthen our foundational values.

In Chapter 7, we will relate the Change and Stability polarity to project-focused change and framework-focused change.

Chapter 7

Project-Focused Change and Framework-Focused Change

I had a call from the head of Organizational Development for a prestigious medical center. He was thrilled with his new position and looked forward to going to work every day. His responsibilities included close collaboration with the leaders from diverse specialty units, and he told me that he had never worked with so many brilliant practitioners and researchers. "There is nothing they can't handle," he explained. "It's a very special place." The medical center is a known exemplar for leading change in our country, and it is already up on most of the problems being talked about in the literature and in frequent health bulletins. "They generally have a plan ready to address the latest issues," he explained, "and whenever changes have to be made there is a great enthusiasm to do whatever is necessary to make it happen."

The medical center's leaders, however, tended to start many initiatives simultaneously. He said that he was hearing the directors express more and more concern about the difficulty people were having keeping all the balls in the air. He, too, was starting to get worried about this pattern.

Over the past 30 years, I have had the privilege of working with many organizations whose leaders are committed, intelligent people desiring to improve the structures and processes of their organizations and the outcomes of the services they render. The need and desire to transform healthcare cultures and practices is not new. I realized many years ago that no matter where our team went, the problems, the concerns, the culture, and the practice issues seemed to be the same everywhere. The important issues revolved around the mission of healthcare systems. I also realized that the nature and intensity of the work at hand was such that we needed one another to be successful. If we could only put our heads together across organizations, states, and countries, we could reach our goals in new and innovative ways.

To make a long story short, there was no such umbrella organization to foster this kind of work in healthcare, so I created one: the Clinical Practice Model Resource Center's (CPMRC) International Consortium. The members of the consortium were drawn together by a shared purpose: to co-create the best places to give and receive care. Each member organization designated a representative to connect to the center, and together we created a learning community with quarterly sessions and a major annual conference. Our work together was driven by the Clinical Practice Model Framework, which provided tools and resources to carry out this collective effort.

One of the frequent problems identified by the CPMRC International Consortium members was the exhaustion related to the numerous projects and initiatives taking place in their own healthcare systems. Many representatives explained that before one project was ended, another one had already launched and it seemed like the staff was always "putting out fires." Consortium representatives were describing their reality, yet they did not think of this as the downside of a polarity. In fact, it took a while for us to figure out what the polarity was called.

We noticed a pattern unfolding when it came to the way institutions dealt with new or troubling situations. Committed leaders understood that at the core of quality healthcare is the ability to identify and solve problems. The "problem" was given a project name and a group or unit committee was assigned to fix the situation. Any process created to address problems had to be strong, so "project management" became a priority. It is no surprise that there was a move to strengthen project management skills across the organization. The good news is that many healthcare professionals are good at project management, which is a very critical skill. Leaders knew that having an efficient and effective approach to address the problems was essential, and project management resulted in many prompt actions to identify and implement actions to address significant problems within healthcare. Yet in the absence of Polarity Thinking, another pattern developed: many project/initiatives worked for a while and then failed over time or were left behind by the beginning of a new project.

We worked hard to break this pattern and soon learned that our framework-driven change model was making a difference in the transformation work in many clinical settings within the consortium. We realized that it was because of the framework-driven change model that we were successful in breaking the pattern. We now understood this fundamental polarity and decided to name it: Project-Driven Change and Framework-Driven Change.

Project-Driven Change and Framework-Driven Change Polarity

Completed Map for Project-Driven Change and Framework-Driven Change Polarity

Greater Purpose Statement (GPS)
Sustainable quality outcomes
Why leverage this polarity?

Action Steps
How will we gain or maintain the positive results from focusing on this left pole? What? Who? By when? Measures?

A. Establish guidelines to identify and act on important point-of-care issues.
B. Provide project management structure, process, financial support, and outcome reporting methods for the teams working on priority practice issues.
C. Use established and known process improvement methods.
D. Engage the key stakeholders and organization's subject-matter experts in the project.

Early Warnings
Measurable indicators (things you can count) that will let you know that you are getting into the downside of this left pole.

A. "Here we go again with another project."
B. "Don't worry, this will go away just like the other initiatives in the past."
C. "We work hard, it improves for a while, and then surprise, not only do things decline, but other problems surface."
D. "We know the details, but nothing is connected."
E. "We use water on the fire but ignore the wind."

Values = positive results from focusing on the left pole
- There is a clear process to help identify and implement projects necessary to improve care and services.
- There is a process to understand all aspects of the problem that needs to be solved.
- Prompt actions are taken to implement projects that improve care and service outcomes.

Values = positive results from focusing on the right pole
- There is consideration of the impact of a change on different parts of the organization.
- The team's input is sought related to the possible impact of the proposed change effort on the organization.
- Change efforts lead to positive sustainable outcomes that support the organization's vision.

Project-Driven Change *and* **Framework-Driven Change**

- Change processes are started before understanding how it might impact all parts of the organization.
- There is a need for "re-work" after changes were made because of unforeseen effects on other areas of the organization.
- The positive results of a change effort are lost because new problems popped up.

Fears = negative results from over-focusing on the left pole *to the neglect of the right pole*

- There is a lack of formal processes or methods to carry out care and service improvement projects.
- There is an inability to promptly identify problems that need to be solved.
- There is an inability to act quickly on care and service projects necessary to improve clinical outcomes.

Fears = negative results from over-focusing on the right pole *to the neglect of the left pole*

Action Steps
How will we gain or maintain the positive results from focusing on this right pole? What? Who? By when? Measures?

A. Establish a process to understand how a framework guides and sustains transformation of practice at the point of care.
B. Ensure change is purpose-driven and guided by mission and core beliefs/values.
C. Know the impact of culture on outcomes.
D. Evaluate the fundamental skills, standards, and infrastructures related to work and critical thinking and reasoning processes.

Early Warnings
Measurable indicators (things you can count) that will let you know that you are getting into the downside of this right pole.

A. "We have so many issues we could improve on if we would only focus on them."
B. "Nothing gets done quickly around here."
C. "We see the forest but not the trees."

Deeper Fear
Unable to sustain quality outcomes
Loss of Greater Purpose

The Project/Framework polarity represents another example of what I call the mother polarities. In its simplicity, it is about the part and the whole. *Project Management* refers to a set of competencies necessary to plan, start, and complete a specific and defined project that has a beginning and an end. A framework approach creates and articulates the bigger picture. When we speak of transforming healthcare, we begin by acknowledging the big-picture "whole" and go from there into the complicated problems that need to be solved within the context of a whole system with many moving parts.

Polarity Thinking makes sense of the exhaustion and frustration occurring within the consortium. We were able to articulate what was happening: our colleagues were in the downside of the Project pole as evidenced by the need for rework, surprising outcomes, and inability to sustain the positive outcomes of a project. They were experiencing the loss of the upsides of the Framework pole.

We soon understood how important it is to have a solid framework to guide our collective work to transform healthcare. Back at the CPMRC, we dove into intense work related to this pole because it was clear that the healthcare systems were becoming more complex and struggling to meet ever-increasing demands. Our present systems had to be transformed into an **integrated healthcare system** across the continuum of care, and to do that, we needed to know more about the whole of reality, especially at the point of care.

The healthcare field has had little or no experience with the framework pole as a guide for large-scale change.

John Naisbitt, a world-renowned futurist, offers his own perspective regarding the importance of having frameworks: "I felt that in a world where events and ideas were analyzed to the point of lifelessness, where complexity grew by quantum leaps, where the information din was so high that one had to shriek to be heard above it, people were hungry for structure. With a simple framework, we could begin to make sense of the world. And we could change the framework as the world itself changed" (2006). He speaks eloquently of the need for a Framework pole.

The members of the CPMRC International Consortium recognized the familiar cycle of going to the downside of the Project pole and its consequences. They concluded that this cycle needed to be broken.

The CPM Framework

The consortium already had a shared purpose to co-create the best places to give and receive care, which naturally became the greater purpose for the Project/Framework polarity. Members were already committed to achieve sustainable transformation in the culture and practices realms that would benefit patients, families, caregivers, and community.

The conceptual underpinnings of the framework, as seen in the figure above, are Core Beliefs, Principles of Dialogue, Partnership and Polarity Thinking and theories, including Systems Thinking, Complexity Science, and Quality and Sociotechnical theory.

In addition, there are six expanding clinical practice models. These models address the underlying assumptions and actions needed to transform both culture and practice, and include an implementation process based on Transformation Science and communities of practice literature. The framework guides the action steps necessary to act within the whole of an extremely complex system. (Lessons from the field are published in the professional literature.)

When there is understanding that each project relates to a greater whole, it brings the action steps to a different level. The framework is a guide to know reality and use that information to address the issues at hand. When there is a commitment of leadership to be guided by a framework and intentions to seek to know the whole, a new set of approaches and questions will emerge that need to be reviewed before any project begins.

Organizations are expected to meet professional standards, credentialing, and governmental controls and will be held accountable for these things. They will have to prepare many documents related to vision, mission, beliefs, values, practice models, processes they support, policy, procedures, etc. Often the former documents are representation of the many projects that were undertaken to produce them. Placing the former within a framework that guides change, by integrating core information, is seldom done. What is written is only as good as it is lived. Commitment to live within the context of the whole takes work and patience.

The action steps to support the Framework pole are:

- Insist that those addressing a problem are clear on the core beliefs and know "what matters most" to the organization. This connects teams around a shared purpose.

- The shared purpose is reflective of the mission and vision of the healthcare organization. The organization must make sure that everyone knows how the shared purpose connects to the project at hand.

Just as understanding the theories related to project management are important to the Project pole so are the fundamental theories that form the Framework pole:

- The fundamental theories include Systems Thinking, Complexity Science, Sociotechnical theories, and Quality theories.

- The fundamental skills and principles of Dialogue, Partnership, and Polarity Thinking are essential to the Framework pole, just as understanding the skills and principles of project management are essential. Dialogue and meaningful conversation is at the core of action to address an issue, as well as Partnership across an interprofessional team.

- There is no single discipline, person, department, specialty, or setting that determines quality care. It takes strong interprofessional partnerships across the team to make a real impact on the work at hand.

Without the skill of Polarity Thinking, the downsides of related poles will continue to emerge. A framework defines the core of our work as healthcare leaders. That is why it exists. It guides, not just with theories but with a commitment to action. It is the move to bring theory to reality, and it must address the desired outcomes.

The framework uses clinical practice models, which support the patient, family, community, and care-givers in order to advance the culture and practice of care. The models guide and sustain healthcare trans-formation. Within a framework, each component is intentionally designed, scalable, evidence-based, out-come-producing, replicable, action-oriented, capacity-building, and technology-enabled. All the models relate in some way to each project and give insights into what questions need to be asked at the project level.

When each project is seen related to the whole, these questions must be asked:

1. Does the project support or does the project interfere with the *how* of achieving sustainable out-comes related to health and healing across the life span and across all settings where healing occurs?

2. Does the project support or does it interfere with the infrastructure and culture to ensure partner-ing relationships?

3. Does the project support or does the project interfere with action steps necessary to achieve inter-professional integration at the point of care?

4. Does the project take action steps that are evidence-based?

5. Does the project use the technology and Informatics support for desired outcomes?

The Framework pole is new and challenging. It depends on clear action steps, including a process to help colleagues understand how it relates to the whole of healthcare and the stated need to develop the skills necessary to integrate it in their work. One of the key strengths of the framework is that it has helped guide the identification of common polarities related to the fundamental elements within the framework. It also guides those working with projects through an assessment as to whether the project or initiative is connected to a problem and/or if it is connected to a common polarity.

The CPMRC International Consortium identified some of the common polarities impacting point-of-care transformation. They are presented in the figure on the following page.

As with any polarity, if the Framework pole is focused on to the neglect of the Project pole, it will lead to the downsides of the pole, which is the loss of the Project pole:

- inadequate processes in place to support projects that are needed to improve care
- inability to keep in touch with the clinical realities
- knowing what is needed to improve care and service
- inability to act promptly

The synergy between the Project-Driven Change and Framework-Driven poles accelerates the ability to grow and sustain positive quality outcomes that neither could reach alone. Because the Framework helps identify the many polarities that exist in healthcare, it enhances the team's awareness of common polarities. It also helps the team understand the importance of asking the question: "Is this a problem to be fixed or a polarity that needs to be managed, or both?" It is the beginning of preventing a misdiagnosis and unintended consequences.

This is an especially important polarity for healthcare professionals because it is key to the simplest of dilemmas involving systems within systems within systems, each affecting the other as well as the whole. I believe the reason our work at the CPMRC and within the International Consortium has been successful and sustainable is because of our ability to leverage this polarity. It is imperative that you and others who lead healthcare transformation understand and learn how to manage this pair of interdependent values in order to achieve positive outcomes that will influence the institution's functional and financial stability.

How the work of transformation is carried out is as important as knowing what the nature of the work actually is. Both require leadership that can leverage the vertical and horizontal polarity discussed in Chapter 8.

Basic Polarities within the Framework

Yin and Yang

INTERPROFESSIONAL INTEGRATION

Acute care - Continuum of care
Task services - Scope of Practice services
Treatment-based service - Preventive-based service
License expectations - Organizational expectations
Task acuity - Professional service acuity
Individual Care and Population Care

Competency

Routine tasks - Scope of Practice
Policy/Procedure - Evidence-based
Memory - Critical thinking
Credential regulation - Professional regulation
Clinician workload - Patient needs
Doing - Caring

Integrated Competency

Individual competency - Integrated competency
Individual - Team
Personal accountability - Holding others accountable

HEALTH INFORMATICS

Paper - Automation
Reference - Embedded
Technology platform - Practice platform
Original - Preconfigured
Platform dictated - Intentionally designed
Process - Outcome
Plan - Implement
Patient needs - Staff needs
Flowsheet/structured note driven - Professional framework

HEALTH AND HEALING

Mission - Margin
Whole person care - Medical care
Individual care - Population care
Patient/customer satisfaction - Provider/staff satisfaction
Individual accountability - Organizational accountability
Government/credential expectations - Administrative expectations
Government/credential expectations - Provider expectations
Administration expectations - Provider expectations
Provider of choice - Employer of choice
Retention - Recruitment
Provider - Payer
Tradition - Innovation
Patient safety - Staff safety
Patient engagement - Provider engagement

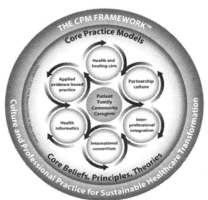

INTERNATIONAL CONSORTIUM

Project - Framework
Local - Global
Change - Stability
Leader - Follower
Teach - Learn

Practice transformation:
Best places to give and
receive care

PARTNERSHIP CULTURE

Communication

Candor - Diplomacy
Listening - Advocacy
Inquiry - Advocacy
Intent - Impact
Talking - Silence

Relationships

Self - Others
Vertical - Horizontal
Conditional respect - Unconditional respect
Productivity - Relationships
Law/consequences - Forgiveness
Justice - Mercy
Confidential - Transparency
Client expectations - Provider expectations
Physician needs - Interdisciplinary needs

Infrastructure

Vertical - Horizontal
Directive decisions - Shared decisions
Centralized - Decentralized
Partnership with colleagues - Partnership with client/families

APPLIED EVIDENCE-BASED PRACTICE

Evidence-based standardized care - Autonomous care
General content - Evidence-based content
Standardized plan of care - Individualized plan of care
Interprofessional education and Interprofessional practice collaboration

Chapter 8

Successful Leaders Leverage Relationship Polarities

The hospital was concerned about the amount of stress at all levels and leadership's inability to engage staff in the work of improving things. There was no sense of ownership. The leaders decided to look at implementing a structure called partnership councils that would bring the staff on the units together to help improve morale. There was a call for volunteers to work on this project, but only a few employees volunteered. A decision was made to pick some people from each unit to learn about the partnership council idea. The workshop participants were discussing the importance of tapping the wisdom of peers when one of the participants said something that brought the group to silence. "I have been here for 20 years", she said, "and this is the first time someone asked me my opinion. It never felt safe to speak up before."

Much has been written about leadership. The polarity map takes the invisible truths about the power of leadership and makes them visible. Parker Palmer—author of *The Courage to Teach* and one of the country's most influential leaders in higher education—described this power eloquently when he said:

> "A leader is a person who has an unusual degree of power to project on other people his or her shadow, or his or her light. A leader is a person who has an unusual degree of power to create the conditions under which other people must live and move and have their being—conditions that can either be as illuminating as heaven or as shadowy as hell."

Polarity helps us understand why some leaders fail and why some are successful. The map and principles of Polarity Thinking give us insights into the importance and impact of power. Understanding this power dynamic makes so many things become clear. The map visualizes the ideal—leaders who inspire, provide hope and direction, and engage the collective in meaningful work. The polarity map reveals the wisdom of such a leader. In the end, successful leaders manage polarities well. They thrive in change because they know change is nothing more than self-corrections in the ongoing oscillation around one or more poles. Organizations whose leaders manage polarities will significantly outperform those that do not.

Leaders who are familiar with polarities know how to remove fear from the work culture. When a problem is presented to them, they know how to dig a little deeper into its origins and identify the polarity below the problem. However, they know something even more important: they know that leadership is about relationships and that *the relationship polarities are the "mother" of all polarities*.

Successful leaders are masters at negotiating not just the vertical relationships, but the horizontal ones. They focus on creating cultures of respect, productivity, and teamwork. They try to involve as many people as possible in the decision-making process and know in their bones that to have a creative, healing, innovative culture that leads to a higher purpose, they must know when there is tension building in one area so they can take immediate action and self-correct. They got where they are because they also know what happens when they take their eyes off the ball.

Polarity Thinking Is Fundamental to Healthy Relationships

Professionals in healthcare management share one fundamental goal: to create the best place to give and receive care, and to grow a healthy, nourishing culture within it that allows everyone to thrive. The majority of adults spend more waking hours at work than they do in their own homes, so the work culture inside our facilities exerts a strong influence on their quality of life as well as those who depend on us.

The work culture reflects the state of relationships within the organization. Healthy relationships involve two or more people who can solve problems and manage ongoing pairs of values (polarities). As with any interdependent pair, there is tension between the two uniquely different individuals. Parker Palmer describes this tension:

> "When we sit in a circle of trust, we are given one experience after another in holding the tension of opposites; experiences that slowly break our hearts open to greater capacity."

The relationship polarities are so important to what we do because being human is all about relationships. Without relationships, there is no humanity. Relationships are about power, individual and collective, but *healthy relationships* call for us to recognize, manage, and treat the tension—the power between two uniquely different individuals—so that quality of life can be achieved. I find that the mapping process in the Polarity Thinking approach provides a picture of the power that exists between humans—individuals and groups. It also shows the power within all the polarities that are evident within human experience.

A Look at the Evolution of Work Relationships

The healthcare systems are historically rooted in hierarchical relationships. Hospitals were often founded by churches, military groups, or academic institutions, all of which are strongly embedded in hierarchical cultures. One of the principles of polarity is to name the two different yet interdependent points of view with neutral names. That is difficult because certain words that are neutral to one person may feel negative to another. Historically in the work culture, relationships were referred to as "boss/subordinate." The boss part of this relationship has often been called hierarchy. Hierarchical relationships are well known in most organizations. For some, hierarchy is a negative term. The reason for that is many individuals have lived in the downside of this pole and have difficulty seeing the positive side of this common word used to describe the pole. Therefore, a more neutral name for some people is to call it vertical relationships. Many organizational charts are vertical. The term *collaboration,* or *partnership,* is seen more positively and can be described as horizontal, showing the opposite or alternative perspective.

The map on the following page illustrates the positive and negative realties of this polarity.

Completed Map for Vertical and Horizontal Relationship Polarity

Greater Purpose Statement (GPS)
Partnerships across the continuum
Why leverage this polarity?

Action Steps
How will we gain or maintain the positive results from focusing on this left pole? What? Who? By when? Measures?

A. Support each person in clarifying professional accountabilities within the scope of practice/services.
B. Provide resources for individuals to independently carry out accountabilities.
C. Provide role clarification and performance criteria.

Values = positive results from focusing on the left pole

- Be clear about your accountability to support the organization's purpose and direction.
- Encourage others to take the initiative to get things done in a timely manner.
- Take pride in your personal contribution to the organization's purpose and direction.

Values = positive results from focusing on the right pole

- The team engages in decision making that impacts the purpose and direction of the organization.
- The team takes ownership for the purpose and direction of the organization.
- The team is proud of their accomplishments that support the purposes and direction of the organization.

Action Steps
How will we gain or maintain the positive results from focusing on this right pole? What? Who? By when? Measures?

A. Establish interdisciplinary partnership infrastructure.
B. Ensure adequate interdisciplinary participation in council sessions.
C. Provide tools and resources that support integrated care across the continuum.
D. Link and connect councils across the continuum of care.
E. Align the purpose and direction of the councils to the organization's direction.

Vertical *and* **Horizontal**

Early Warnings
Measurable indicators (things you can count) that will let you know that you are getting into the downside of this left pole.

A. "It really does not matter what I think around here."
B. "There is a we/they mentality around here."
C. "The culture is one of gossip, blame, and rumors."
D. "It is not my job. Let the bigwigs handle it. That is what they get paid for."
E. "The leadership does not have a clue of what we are dealing with at the bedside."

- There is a failure to use the collective wisdom of the team to further the purpose and direction of the organization.
- There is lack of opportunity for the team to work together to improve care and services.
- There is an inability to work together as a team, preventing a sense of team accomplishment.

Fears = negative results from over-focusing on the left pole *to the neglect of the right pole*

- It is difficult to connect to the greater purpose and direction of the organization.
- There is limited individual freedom to act in a timely manner to improve care or service.
- Individual contributions to the organization go unrecognized.

Fears = negative results from over-focusing on the right pole *to the neglect of the left pole*

Early Warnings
Measurable indicators (things you can count) that will let you know that you are getting into the downside of this right pole.

A. "It is hard to get things done around here... we are spinning our wheels."
B. "Someone needs to make a decision."
C. "Nobody is accountable around here."

Deeper Fear
Lack of partnerships across the continuum
Loss of Greater Purpose

Reflections on the Vertical and Horizontal Relationship Polarity

Are healthcare settings immune to hierarchy? Best practices in healthcare organizations call for individual practitioners who have impeccable abilities to diagnose and treat, as well as find the problem and solve it or fix it. The best practices call for individuals to be clear, knowledgeable, accountable, and decisive. They must be prepared to take action immediately in urgent situations. The healthcare industry is filled with individuals who understand the value, importance, and benefits of the upsides of the Vertical pole, which gives them a sense of accomplishment and importance.

The profession is filled with people who are strong problem solvers and value their own individual power and freedom. Certain job roles call for people who can solve serious problems and make life or death decisions, so it is no coincidence that hospital executives, physicians, managers, and more experienced employees become the people with power. They are champions for this important pole. However, the power becomes "power-over" because there is no balance with the other pole. Because of the dominance of the hierarchy pole and the neglect of the partnership pole, many who practice in healthcare live in the downside of hierarchy.

Remember: *The power dynamic is central to polarity.* People least likely to be concerned about the dynamic are those who hold a lot of power. When a person is imposing his/her pole, he/she does not feel the tension. The outcome of focusing on one pole to the neglect of the other is 100% predictable, and this polarity historically has not been managed well in healthcare.

Healthcare Professionals Recognize this Polarity

This polarity often shows up in the form of complaints and cultures with poor morale, disengagement, and dissatisfaction. The literature describes the silos in healthcare, low morale, powerlessness, and lack of healing relationships among healthcare providers and the people they give care to. Common expressions are heard such as, "No one cares what I think, my opinion doesn't matter. I just do what they say, can't do anything about it. No one tells you what is going on around here." Why are these complaints so common and strong? These are *early warnings* that many of the providers are living in the downside of the Vertical/Hierarchy pole because the Horizontal/Partnership pole is being neglected. The gap of trust between leadership and staff will grow if this polarity is not leveraged well.

Those who live in the downside of hierarchy feel voiceless and not valued. The late poet Maya Angelou wrote about disenfranchisement and its impact on relationships and explained it poignantly:

> "People will forget what you said, people will forget what you did, but people will never forget how you made them feel."

When people feel undervalued or disrespected, they tend to become passive or reactive and resistant. Negativity and confrontation are destructive to organizations and human relationships.

The outcome. The healthcare system as a whole is under fire. Reports and studies from such respected organizations as the American Nurses Association, the American Medical Association, the Volunteer Hospital Association, and the American Association of Nurse Executives indicate that they are focusing on the new realities. So are patient groups. The silos and disconnects across the healthcare system are interfering with the quality of patient care and the quality of the practice for those giving care. Repetition, duplication, omission, and fragmentation within our organizations and facilities are wasting money and resources, but *they are also damaging patient and staff satisfaction.* Staff accountability and engagement in all aspects of care are essential in order to continuously improve. No one person, role, discipline, or department will be able to address the practice issues and care improvements unless there is ownership and creativity at the point of care by all. This cannot be done without collaboration or partnership—the Horizontal/Partnership pole.

When we think about our challenges in terms of interdependency, we can see that there is a need to focus on partnerships and teamwork. It is a natural flow to move toward partnership, because each voice is heard and valued equally, whether it is from provider to provider, provider to manager, or provider to employees, patients, and families.

Collaborating and instilling a sense of *ownership* improves the lives of those who give care and those who receive care. It is hard to believe that if you put all your energy into strengthening team collaboration/partnerships in order to avoid repetition, silos, staff feelings of powerlessness, and so on (thinking perhaps that you can get to manage the hierarchical relationships later), you will still get negative consequences, leading to deeper problems. When an organization is shifting from a hierarchical to collaborative mindset, it is natural to focus only on the promise of partnership. That, however, is not the first step; the first step when managing polarities is to ensure that the most common Hierarchical pole is supported. It is not a comfortable thing to do. The greater purpose of healthier cultures and interprofessional partnership across the continuum needs the synergy of both the Vertical and Horizontal poles.

Why is the hierarchical pole so difficult to manage? The individuals who have power generally believe that all is well. Because this is their dominant point of view, it is difficult for them to know the downside of hierarchical structures. Even when they agree that it would be good to have more "ownership" and collaboration, they still show some resistance. Yes, they value hierarchy, but they have a deeper fear that if this collaborative partnership philosophy takes over, nothing will get done in a timely manner, no one will take accountability, they will lose their individual freedom, and their unique expertise will be lost or not appreciated. Sound familiar? This is also true for clinicians, managers, and executives.

We have all experienced strong Vertical/Hierchary infrastructures in the health-care system, but many do not have a parallel Horizontal/Partnership infrastructure. For a team to work together, there must be an intentionally designed infrastructure embedded into the culture that brings the teams together to do their work and a guarantee that the tools and resources needed to support the relationships necessary to achieve integrated service will be there when they are needed. Unfortunately, departments and indeed many disciplines lack ongoing support and mandates to come together, break down the silos, and learn how to integrate their expertise in an ongoing manner. These committed healthcare providers need new skills to help them develop and nurture sustained partnerships, have meaningful dialogue with integrated teams, and work through difficult conversations.

Understanding fear and distrust. Those who have never been in positions of hierarchical power—and especially those who have lived in the downside of hierarchy—often do not trust people who value hierarchy. They do not have an understanding of hierarchy or an appreciation that those who know the strengths of hierarchy have some legitimate fears about the downside of the Horizontal pole. The people who believe in horizontal structures alternatively are blind to its downsides (especially if they see partnership as a solution). This is what leads to power struggles where there will be no winners.

Clearly, no matter what the healthcare polarity pairs are, those who favor one pole over the other will have strong fears about the other pole. Each group is mistaking its own point of view for the whole. There is no natural tendency to tolerate the work necessary to strengthen the opposite pole. Sharing one's point of view without the awareness that it is only half the truth is perpetuating ignorance of the whole. Effective leaders know their biases and limitations, and will seek the other point of view.

Because there is such a steep learning curve for the skills needed for successful partnership, it is critical for those in hierarchy to be patient, because they will experience the downside of the partnership polarity as they learn.

What will help you leverage this relationship polarity? Recognize the positive attributes of the traditionally dominant Vertical/Hierarchy pole and be sure you do what you must to lower any natural resistance, especially when the Partnership pole is the focus. Be sure to pay attention to the early warnings that show the Vertical/Hierarchy pole is being neglected (e.g., such as individuals are not being supported in the development and delivery of their unique contributions or being acknowledged for them, and decisions are not being made in a timely manner that impact each person's responsibilities whether they are in practice, management, education, or research).

Everyone must understand that individual hierarchical power is an essential element of competency and accountability. Initiate dialogue and share examples of its advantages, such as situations where a patient is in cardiac arrest, it is important for a knowledgeable provider to step in and take the lead. Without that lead person the patient is at risk.

Help those who fear the power of hierarchy know the difference between hierarchy as power-over and hierarchy in synchrony with partnership. Help them see it is not letting go of Vertical/Hierarchy but supplementing it.

Every organization must provide the resources to support the building of a Horizontal/Partnership structure across the organization. The CPMRC International Consortium has been implementing such infrastructure over the past 30 years. These partnership councils spark staff engagement and ownership, but implementation must be done carefully and deliberately because partnership structures do not look like vertical organizational charts and processes, as can be seen in the illustration on the following page.

Horizontal/Partnership Infrastructure

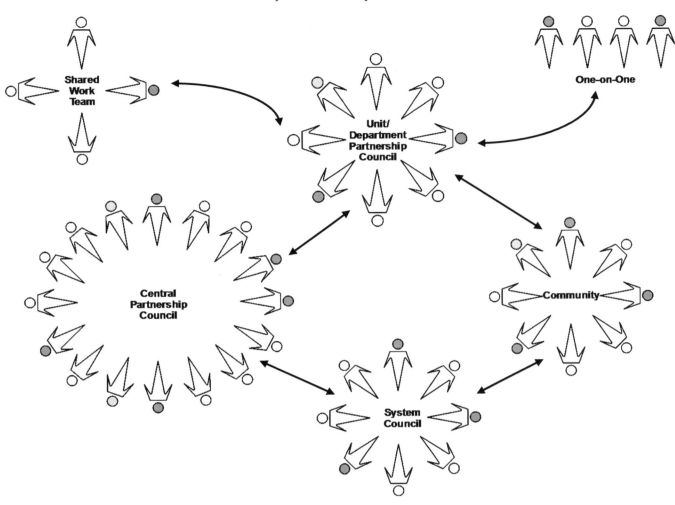

The Vertical and Horizontal Relationship Polarity is only one of the Relationship value pairs. Another one fundamental to great leadership is a pair we refer to as Conditional and Unconditional Respect.

The Conditional Respect and Unconditional Respect Polarity

Respect is a word rooted in our internal beliefs about the value of another human being. It is a word used to describe the fundamental nature of a relationship with another human being. The American Heritage College Dictionary defines *respect* as "to feel or show esteem for, avoid violation of; treat with deference." Respect is not a one-time act but a way of life. It is a valued principle. Respect has two poles: Conditional and Unconditional. One is not more important than the other—both are necessary to create a healthy culture of relationships. A close look at the nature of this polarity and the work to manage it gives insights into the culture of healthcare, an important challenge for all leaders. A completed map for Conditional and Unconditional Respect is presented on the following page.

Completed Map for Conditional Respect and Unconditional Respect Polarity

Greater Purpose Statement (GPS)
A culture of respect
Why leverage this polarity?

Action Steps
How will we gain or maintain the positive results from focusing on this left pole? What? Who? By when? Measures?

A. Assure all are given opportunities to develop skills related to standards of care/service.
B. Provide current job descriptions with clear and achievable performance measures.
C. Assure that orientation and continuous learning opportunities support practice/service standards and competencies.
D. Assure updated and objective performance evaluation tools are in place.
E. Celebrate successful skill development.

Values = positive results from focusing on the left pole

- Everyone is clear about role, expectations, goals, policies, procedures, evidence-based practice, and performance measurements
- People feel respected and supported for what they do well
- Individuals are responsible, accountable, and self-confident in their contributions
- Expertise is developed and grown through diverse learning

Values = positive results from focusing on the right pole

- There is value for each person as an authentic human being regardless of status, job description, education level, or performance
- Peers mentor and support desiring their success
- Creates safe place to share perspectives
- Listened to with great attention
- Engaged in decision making
- Involved in self-growth and learning, which invites trying new things

Action Steps
How will we gain or maintain the positive results from focusing on this right pole? What? Who? By when? Measures?

A. Create opportunities to develop/enhance the skills of partnership, dialogue, and Polarity Management
B. There is an expectation within the organization that we honor each person's unique story, know their values, and professional and personal strengths
C. The organizational culture supports the elements of being the best place to give and receive care
D. Provide tools and resources to support the competency of each person, both in doing (actions) and being (individuality), art and science

Conditional Respect *and* **Unconditional Respect**

Early Warnings
Measurable indicators (things you can count) that will let you know that you are getting into the downside of this left pole.

A. "This is how we do it here."
B. "It's all about what you do, not who you are or can be."
C. "This relationship stuff is nothing but fluff."
D. "We are afraid of doing something wrong because no one ever forgets about it."
E. "You make a mistake here, you will hear about it."

- Individuals only feel valued for what they do as defined by the organization or peers
- Restrictive and punitive environment leads to fear, coverups, and inaccurate information
- Loss of individuality: do not feel respected, valued, or listened to
- Just play the game, conform, and decrease risk-taking and innovation

Fears = negative results from over-focusing on the left pole *to the neglect* of the right pole

- Not clear about role, expectations, goals, policies, procedures, evidence-based practice, and performance measurement
- Lack of individual and collective accountability for contribution
- Tolerance for poor performance even when it causes errors
- Lack of self-awareness to improve and enhance accomplishments and learning

Fears = negative results from over-focusing on the right pole *to the neglect* of the left pole

Early Warnings
Measurable indicators (things you can count) that will let you know that you are getting into the downside of this right pole.

A. "Everybody is nice, but nobody is helping me be a better clinician."
B. There is an increase in complaints, errors, and variance, but no one talks about it.
C. There is a drop in performance measures/standards.
D. There is a decrease in teaching/learning programs.

Deeper Fear
Unable to sustain a culture of respect
Loss of Greater Purpose

Reflections on the Conditional Respect and Unconditional Respect Polarity

Conditional Respect

The conditional respect pole is critical to the mission of healthcare. Quality healthcare depends on the expertise of diverse members of the healthcare team. It is essential that each person is competent and is becoming more competent all the time. It is their ability "to perform" that generates deep conditional respect. That explains why the conditional pole has been dominant in healthcare. Specific action steps have been taken to keep this pole strong such as listing the responsibilities and describing the skills that demonstrate competency in job descriptions, orientation programs, continuous learning opportunities, policies, procedures, and standards of care. In addition, often a preceptor works side by side with new people to evaluate the listed competency before getting off orientation.

However, when this pole is focused on at the neglect of Unconditional Respect, the early warnings will appear such as comments like "What rules here is," "This is how we do it here," "The only thing that matters is what you do, not who you are or can be," "There is a lot of fear because no one ever forgets if you do something wrong." The consequence of over-focusing on Conditional Respect is that the culture becomes negative and dehumanized.

Actions to Strengthen Unconditional Respect

Actions to support Unconditional Respect require the principles of Partnership, Dialogue, and Polarity Thinking to be taught and used by the whole team. Unconditional Respect requires that each person is listened to and recognized for the unique contributions they bring. They are listened to as a person with a head on their shoulders, a heart in their chest, and unique perspectives and interests worthy of attention from those they work for and with. Orientation looks different because it evolves around knowing the individual's story, strengths, and weaknesses and demonstrating accountability to help them become successful. As a valued member of the team, their success is everyone's success. Sometimes in the hectic activities of the day, it is hard to believe the time spent with someone you don't care for or who is less educated, less experienced, with very different perspectives can make a positive difference to the work at hand.

The Downsides of Relationships

Successful leaders in the healthcare field do whatever they can to manage relationships and partnerships. If they fail at this, the organization's culture starts to deteriorate. When employees feel powerless, good leaders find out about it and reach out to balance the power and raise staff morale. When people feel disrespected and believe that they have no "voice," the dissatisfaction and frustration grow into a pressing need to change the circumstances. A great deal of discord and broken faith in the institution and its management comes from such perceived betrayal. Polarity maps illustrate this aspect of the power/relationship dynamic.

The words used to describe the power within relationships might vary, but the underlying principles of power balance between two or more people are always the same. There is no power without relationships, because "power" represents a pattern in a relationship. Jim Rohn, a personal development consultant and motivational speaker, said this about leadership:

> "The challenge of leadership is to be strong, but not rude; be kind, but not weak; be bold, but not bully; be thoughtful, but not lazy; be humble, but not timid; be proud, but not arrogant; have humor, but without folly."

Polarity Thinking teaches one how to do that. It helps leaders see the presence of power and the impact of power in their organizations. In the next chapter, we look at an additional relationship polarity and its impact on unionization.

Chapter 9

Unionization Efforts and Organizational Relationships

The nurses in the hospital decided to go on strike because of the heavy workload, the stressful culture, and inadequate pay. Many of the hospitals in the state were unionized, but this particular hospital's strike received a lot of attention because this was one of the longest strikes in state history—and there was physical violence. The managers admitted that they were fearful of their safety. The animosity was palpable—each side was fighting for power. The contractual process was the focus by both sides. One leader was reported to have said, "I don't think it will ever be better. Three of us are planning on leaving. I think this is hopeless."

When we get a bit closer to the human story behind an employee strike, we see that there are sincere people on both sides who feel disenfranchised and conflicted about what is happening. They seem like reasonable people with legitimate concerns, yet the public spectacle is sometimes too emotional and scary. *How did things get to this point?* we ask ourselves. The Polarity Thinking approach is particularly relevant in such circumstances, because it allows us to hold true to our views without fear or resentment *and* we can now see the truths behind the other side's position. It takes away the need to spend so much energy trying to convince everyone else to think like we do. Thinking of relationships as polarities and illustrating their dynamics allows us to remember the different kinds of relationships in our own lives. We can then put together a set of principles related to the power within relationships. This chapter will focus on work cultures that are either union or non-union and how we can leverage their strengths and possibilities. We sometimes refer to the polarity pair as the Covenant and Contract Relationships polarity.

Some Historical Context

There are two well-known authors/leaders who have spoken or written about this polarity. The first was the Russian writer and critic of Soviet totalitarianism, Aleksandr Solzhenitsyn. About the subject, Solzhenitsyn wrote this:

> "A society which is based on the letter of the law and never reaches any higher is taking very scarce advantage of the high level of human possibilities. The letter of the law is too cold and formal to have a beneficial effect on society. Whenever the tissue of life is woven of legalistic relationships, there is an atmosphere of moral mediocrity, paralyzing man's noblest impulses."

It is clear that Solzhenitsyn is referring to the loss, the lower right quadrant, of the Covenant relationships pole. We can place his statement on the map below in the lower right quadrant.

Max De Pree, author of *Leadership Is an Art* and *Leadership Jazz*, is known for his leadership philosophy and belief in open communication and inclusiveness within organizations. He states:

> "Covenant relationships are vastly different from Contracts. They deal in shared beliefs, shared values, shared commitments, and shared promises... exhibit love and commitment together in the pursuit of our mission. It means that we spend reflective time together; that we're vulnerable to each other; that we can challenge each other in love and deal with conflicts as mature adults."

De Pree is obviously talking about the value, the upper left quadrant, of a relationship polarity called Covenant. We can place his statement on the map below in the upper left quadrant.

Diagonals of the Covenant Relationships Pole

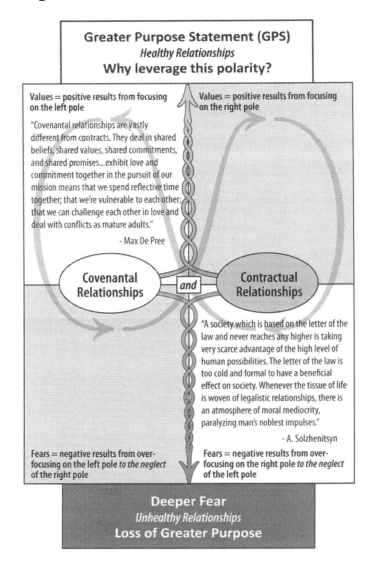

The process of incorporating both leaders' views on a map helps us understand this important interdependent polarity pair. Clearly, the preference pole for both leaders is the Covenant pole. Remember: a pole represents the values of the pole and the fear of losing the values. Preference poles have a strong positive association with one pole and a fear of the downside of the other pole. Max De Pree described the upside of Covenant relationships and Aleksandr Solzhenitsyn described the downside of contract relationships (or the loss of the upsides of covenant relationships). When we map the comments, it becomes apparent that we are missing some information and the picture is incomplete. The content within the map has taken the spirit of their comments and placed it in outcome language.

Both leaders, living decades apart, were interested in the power that exists within relationships. In a conversation about relationships, it is rare to hear people talk about them as parts of a pair of opposites, but that is precisely what is important here.

Completed Map for Covenant and Contract Relationships Polarity

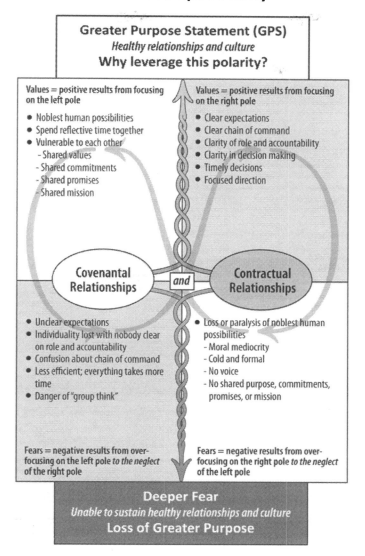

Greater Purpose Statement (GPS)
Healthy relationships and culture
Why leverage this polarity?

Values = positive results from focusing on the left pole

- Noblest human possibilities
- Spend reflective time together
- Vulnerable to each other
  - Shared values
  - Shared commitments
  - Shared promises
  - Shared mission

Values = positive results from focusing on the right pole

- Clear expectations
- Clear chain of command
- Clarity of role and accountability
- Clarity in decision making
- Timely decisions
- Focused direction

Covenantal Relationships *and* **Contractual Relationships**

- Unclear expectations
- Individuality lost with nobody clear on role and accountability
- Confusion about chain of command
- Less efficient; everything takes more time
- Danger of "group think"

- Loss or paralysis of noblest human possibilities
  - Moral mediocrity
  - Cold and formal
  - No voice
  - No shared purpose, commitments, promises, or mission

Fears = negative results from over-focusing on the left pole *to the neglect* of the right pole

Fears = negative results from over-focusing on the right pole *to the neglect* of the left pole

Deeper Fear
Unable to sustain healthy relationships and culture
Loss of Greater Purpose

Notice how their perspectives connect with one another when placed on a map. Solzhenitsyn lived in a society dominated by contract/legalistic relationships and lived in its downside. De Pree spoke to the upside of the Covenant pole. Neither man referred to the positives of a Contract pole nor the downsides of the Covenant pole. Nevertheless, they were clearly letting their readers know their preference. They did not frame their beliefs in terms of a polarity or call them such, but it is clear that they were focusing on the Covenant pole.

The benefits that come when the preferred pole is managed well will be lost if equal attention is not paid to the Contract pole (which exists and must be addressed). Contract relationships are often a part of employment, credentialing, and professional and financial realities. Those in negotiations know the power of both. We have two famous leaders speaking to the importance of relationships and acknowledging the Covenant and Contract Relationships polarity, yet not making the tacit wisdom of the other pole visible. What is important here is that over time they will experience unintended consequences if they are unaware that their views are part of a polarity. The map makes the tacit wisdom obvious and prevents seeing either pole as a solution. Without knowing about polarities, it becomes a fight to win, and in that war, all will lose in the end.

If any polarity is not being managed well, it will show up in various ways, **including agitation and avoidance in the form of complaints, conflicts, and resistance to change.**

The effort to unionize is essentially an attempt to address the imbalance of power that exists within human relationships. When employees have a sense of powerlessness, they will reach out to balance the power and take action to change the circumstances. Most of the problems that lead to unionization efforts exist as the result of dominant unipolar thinking related to the common polarities that exist in healthcare. The preference poles of those people who hold the power are dominant. Everybody else stands somewhere along the downside of that pole.

There are many polarities not being managed well in healthcare, but it is the relationship polarities that will drive the unionization movement. The lack of respect, decision making, and inclusiveness, among other things, will drive unionization efforts.

Most conflicts within healthcare are the result of an imbalance of power between employer and employee, administration/manager and staff, provider and provider, staff and staff, one discipline and another discipline, provider and person/family receiving care, physicians and administration, physicians and nurses, hospital and payers, etc. The imbalance can be present at many levels.

Most clinical settings have operated within cultures favoring Vertical over Horizontal, Conditional Respect over Unconditional Respect, or Contractual relationship over Covenant. This unipolar dominance explains the frustration that leads those living in the downside to call for help. When there is unequal power coupled by a strong *either/or* mindset, regardless of the circumstances, failure is 100% predictable over time because one pole is being neglected.

People who work in the downside of the employer's preferred polarity have three options:

1. They can remain powerless and depend on the benevolence of organizational leadership.

2. They can lobby and even beg the people with the power to be benevolent and do the right thing for their employees.

3. They can figure out a way to gain some power from the employer's pole.

The major problem is seeing it as *either/or* because it then turns into a power struggle that one side needs to win. *Either/or* is coming from both sides. The hope sits in the concept of shared power. When someone has the power, shared power can be very uncomfortable. Polarity Thinking is about shared power in the sense that both poles together generate *more* power. From a polarity perspective, sharing power enhances one's power. The relationship polarities are about the freedom to bring multiple voices together in order to understand the whole of a complex reality. This creates a safe environment for those who give and receive care.

The question I have asked often is, What would our cultures look like today, if from the beginning of the healthcare system formation, the logic of Polarity Thinking (both/and) was the norm? We do know the outcomes, the downsides, when there is an absence of this missing logic.

Chapter 10

Why Many Safety Efforts Have Cost Millions and Are Not Sustainable

When the Institute of Medicine declared over ten years ago that the U.S. healthcare industry had some serious safety issues that needed to be addressed, the response by healthcare leaders was immediate. We had a problem that needed to be fixed and prioritized as soon as possible.

Each of us possesses a deep need to feel safe. The healthcare system has always valued safety. It is the essence of our practice. We prevent, heal, help, and we "do no harm." However, because of the recent complex realities within our healthcare system, the reports of unsafe hospital or care situations has taken center stage.

The Institute of Medicine reports highlight major safety problems, such as medication errors, failure to prevent complications, failure to rescue, inability to stop duplication repetition and omissions, and the lack of tools and evidence-based resources and organizational infrastructures to enhance team integration across the continuum.

Healthcare providers know that the work around safety is very important and worthy of the time and energy needed to address the safety deficiencies. Yet for all the work and the millions of dollars still being spent on safety, the outcomes are still not as good as desired and are often not sustainable. A 2011 report of a ten-year study of efforts to improve cost, quality, and safety within the nation's healthcare system noted that overall adverse events were not decreasing—they were going up! One-third of hospital patients admitted for care experienced adverse events. One-third!

There are dozens of diverse problems that come under the umbrella of safety, and you can undoubtedly come up with long lists from your own experience. However, underneath the many problems that make the environment unsafe are values that must be strengthened and leveraged. The framework used in the Polarity Thinking approach provides insights into the many polarities that relate to safety (see Chapter 7).

If a safety concern is brought to light by a credentialing body, the media, articles in professional journals, or reports from national medical committees such as the Institute of Medicine, the best healthcare organizations respond in a flurry. The first pattern of response is to let the public know that the organization believes the problem is serious and important, that it is doing something about it, and that everyone within the organization is on alert. A good example is the response to the Ebola crisis.

The next step is predictable. The issue is destined to be assigned its own committee. After the Institute's 1999 report, safety committees were set up across the country. Then what? Safety is seen as a problem that will be fixed. The public is reassured that such a committed group will figure it out and make us all safe again. The ownership sits with those on the committee who have time to meet, discuss, evaluate, and report. There is great fervor around the issue, and when a problem is met with fervor in healthcare, another pattern arises.

When the committee is named and begins its work, someone comes up with a slogan for the important issue at hand. This slogan becomes the name of the new project plan designed to solve the problem. An example: the committee working on the restraint saga picked the slogan: "No Restraints on Patient Safety." There is energy and pride around this snappy concise statement, and everyone thinks that it will inspire and engage the rest of the people in the organization to buy in to this worthy effort.

Once a safety issue is raised to the slogan status, another pattern emerges. The new slogan gets a lot of attention initially, but eventually it will be left behind and replaced by another slogan for a more pressing problem, but it will resurface later.

Since we have lived through the major fervor around restraints and the aftermath of the decisions, what might we learn that will give us insights related to safety as a greater purpose?

Thousands of hours of discussions were held across the country on the topic of restraints and thousands of dollars were spent on new forms, elaborate processes, and new procedures and protocols within hospital settings to address the restraint issue.

Organizational leaders and committees worried that their facilities would not meet the new restraint standards, so they created safety committees and new elaborate forms, policies, and procedures and often without provider involvement. When they hear that there is staff resistance, they are caught off-guard. *But the cause is so honorable! How can there be any resistance? Don't they know what we are doing?*

Why *shouldn't* there be resistance? No policies, procedures, and protocols will be complete or effective if the other pole is not supported. If these safety committees had understood at the outset that every safety deficiency is part of an underlying polarity, they could have rejected approaches and presented new possibilities to help ensure sustainable interventions.

In a 2000 article on restraints appearing in the *Journal of Health Care Law and Policy*, authors Braun and Capezuti noted this: "No clinical study demonstrates that any intervention, including restraints, unequivocally prevents falls or fall-related injuries, a major safety issue. In fact, one half of all falls occur among restrained residents and serious injury rates are higher in facilities that use restraints. The underlying issue is *fall risk*. The routine restraint use does not constitute good legal risk management... *The real basis of liability is a lack of Care (by provider) to address fall risk.*"

In the end, we are down to a very important point: healthcare patients and the staff of the facility are interconnected. This is a core polarity, and it raises a question: What are the polarities associated with the greater purpose of Safety for those who give care *and* for those who receive care? It begins with a basic polarity of Patient Safety and Staff Safety.

Completed Map for the Patient Safety and Staff Safety Polarity

Greater Purpose Statement (GPS)
A culture of safety for both those who give and receive care
Why leverage this polarity?

Action Steps
How will we gain or maintain the positive results from focusing on this left pole? What? Who? By when? Measures?

A. Ensure there is a process to obtain the patient's story, body, mind, and spirit.
B. Establish an integrated team to synchronize care mutually with the patient.
C. Integrate evidence-based literature into the decision making regarding patient safety.
D. Care process involves partnerships being established with patients, family, and team.
E. Review and create action plans based on the findings of incident reports.
F. Utilize methods to promote patient safety such as "stop the line," etc.
G. Implement interprofessional plan of care process across the continuum.

Early Warnings
Measurable indicators (things you can count) that will let you know that you are getting into the downside of this left pole.

A. Staff complain of inadequate resources to support giving safe care.
B. Staff complain that there is no time to provide safe individualized care.
C. Staff complain about not feeling safe in their roles or assignments.
D. "It is hard to keep the patient safe when I do not have what I need to do my work."
E. "There are so many patient safety regulations that they are preventing me from giving safe care."

Values = positive results from focusing on the left pole

- Patients and family openly express their needs.
- The team involves the patients and families as partners to improve care and services.
- Care and services are given to help patients and families understand and find meaning in their health situation.

Patient Safety *and* **Staff Safety**

- There is a lack of evidence-based resources to support staff in the delivery of safe care.
- The work environment is unsafe for staff.
- The workload interferes with the ability of staff to provide safe care.

Fears = negative results from over-focusing on the left pole *to the neglect* of the right pole

Values = positive results from focusing on the right pole

- There are adequate evidence-based resources necessary for staff to deliver safe care and services.
- There is a safe work environment for staff.
- Working conditions are structured to support the staff in the delivery of safe care.

- Patients and families lack the opportunity to express their individual needs.
- Patients and families have little control over their care and services.
- Staff are unable to help patients and families find meaning in their health situation.

Fears = negative results from over-focusing on the right pole *to the neglect* of the left pole

Action Steps
How will we gain or maintain the positive results from focusing on this right pole? What? Who? By when? Measures?

A. Provide tools and resources necessary to carry out professional practice/service safely.
B. Establish interdisciplinary partnership infrastructures to facilitate coordination of care.
C. Ensure evidence-based information is available to support delivery of care.
D. Create a culture of safety.
E. The organization involves staff in their evaluation and mitigation of environmental risks.
F. Ensure adequate time and assignment to support professional processes.

Early Warnings
Measurable indicators (things you can count) that will let you know that you are getting into the downside of this right pole.

A. Patients complain about not feeling safe or cared for.
B. Patients feel like just another number.
C. Patients complain about getting contradictory information from the team, which makes them feel unsafe.
D. "No one seems to know what is going on. I get a different story with each caregiver."
E. There is a decrease in submission of patient incident reports by staff.

Deeper Fear
Unable to create a culture of safety for both those who give and receive care
Loss of Greater Purpose

Reflections on Patient Safety and Staff Safety Polarity

Upsides. The map spells out critical outcomes that healthcare providers value for each pole. With the Patient Safety pole, the desired outcomes include patients/families feeling safe and comfortable in expressing their needs. They will work in partnership with the staff to improve care, and they will understand and find meaning in their health situation. The desired outcomes for the Staff Safety pole include having all the necessary evidence-based resources needed in order to provide safe care, and having a safe environment that is structured specifically so that they can provide quality care.

Over-focusing on patient safety. What happens when the focus is on Patient Safety at the neglect of Staff Safety? There are early warnings that will surface, such as staff complaints: "It's hard to keep patients safe when I do not have what I need to do my work, when I am not feeling safe in my assignment or role, or when there are so many patient-safety regulations that prevent me from giving safe care."

The early warnings are meant to show everyone that staff members are experiencing the downsides of the Patient Safety pole, which is the loss of the upsides of the Staff Safety pole. This suggests that there is a need to support the action steps for Staff Safety. The action steps are not quick fixes and are often new to many organizations (e.g., providing evidence-based tools and resources for each of the interdisciplinary teams; providing infrastructures for teams to coordinate care; involving staff in decisions to mitigate environmental risks; and making sure assignments are safe). These are very different action steps than those that strengthen and improve patient safety.

Over-focusing on staff safety. What happens when the focus is on staff safety to the neglect of patient safety? There are early warnings (e.g., Patients and families are complaining about not feeling safe or cared for. They feel like another number. They get contradictory information and are not sure what is going on). Action steps that would change this might include coming up with a definitive process that begins every care regime with knowing the patient's story (body, mind, and spirit). Then there must be an integrated team to synchronize care in partnership with the patient/family to create an evidence-based, individualized plan of care.

Polarity Thinking teaches us that when the downsides are felt, it is because the action steps already spelled out *are not being taken or do not go far enough.* When a polarity is recognized, the approach to address it changes, so the stakeholders have to then decide what action steps need to be taken in their organization for both poles.

Action steps. The content of the maps in this book represent some of the most common positive and negative behaviors and desired outcomes and action steps and early warnings related to common healthcare polarities. The CPMRC's International Consortium has identified patterns of actions steps that have strengthened the interdependent polarity pairs in their organizations. Each organization simply needs to have the conversation as to what they *must* do to strengthen each pole, based on their situation. In fact, many of the action steps listed throughout this book emerged as consensus priorities. The information in the maps is not meant to include every possible circumstance, but rather to provide some priority information for all components of the map.

This chapter has presented the broad polarity of Patient Safety and Staff Safety. This is just the beginning. The Institute of Medicine's 2004 report noted this: "...reducing error and increasing patient safety are not likely to be achieved by any single action, but a comprehensive approach addressing all components of healthcare delivery within an organization is required."

The work around safety never ends, because the polarities related to safety are unstoppable, unavoidable, unsolvable, and indestructible. The greater purpose of a culture of safety calls for vigilance to make sure that the many related polarities and specific problems are managed well. Safety is rooted in the way we practice and in every component of the whole care process within the organization as well as the clinical setting. The variables are numerous. Our goal is to continuously improve the care we give. Therefore, we will continuously be faced with newly diagnosed interdependent pairs and new problems that I hope will help us reach a greater purpose not even imagined today.

Additional polarities related to safety. This chapter has presented the broad example of Patient Safety and Staff Safety, but there are other specific polarities that are related to safety, such as Task and Scope of Practice; Evidence-Based Standardized Care and Autonomous Care; Individual Competency and Integrated Competency; Directive and Shared Decision Making; and Productivity and Relationships all covered in Section Two. When you look at the downsides of these polarities, it becomes very clear that they are part of the overall culture of safety. Keeping people safe is one of our most important goals as healthcare practitioners and leaders. Polarity Thinking honors our natural human fears by making them transparent and by teaching us how to control them in order to live securely in the face of those fears.

Polarity Thinking eliminates the paralysis of fear and creates an oscillation that manages the situation so that we know how to make sure that those legitimate fears do not become reality.

Problems related to safety will continue to surface, demanding us to take prompt action. The next chapter will address how Polarity Thinking provides direction as we seek to comply with safety-related mandates on every level.

Chapter 11

Mandates: Electronic Healthcare Record and Practice Platform

The room was filled with executives from dozens of organizations that had purchased the same Electronic Health Record software platform. One of the CEOs explained how her organization implemented the system. The outcomes were impressive. The chief information officer for a different organization stood up and said, "I have purchased the exact same system that you have, with all the same intensions to improve the care at the bedside. We have not achieved any of the outcomes you have described. How is that possible?"

Leaders in healthcare are faced with many internal and external mandates that must be met at multiple levels. Mandated change is generally driven by government, credentialing bodies, or financial incentives. The federal mandate to implement the Electronic Health Record (EHR) demonstrates the importance of Polarity Thinking when any mandate is given. That is why we devote this chapter to the subject.

Historically, mandates were seen by organizations as problems that must be addressed. That is what happened with the EHR mandate. When the American Recovery and Reinvestment Act (known as the Stimulus program) was passed by Congress in 2009, it allocated billions of dollars to the healthcare industry to help address two main problems facing the healthcare system: the growing cost of healthcare, and the concern for the safety and quality of care for all of society throughout their life span. In the years since, the focus on safety, quality, and cost-containment has shifted to point of care, where the hands of those who give and the hands of those who receive care meet. The goal to improve clinical outcomes is about the realities of practice. However, the focus on the EHR mandate is about technology.

Mandates are often seen as solutions to a problem that needs to be addressed. That approach was true for many organizations that implemented the EHR system. The result: After billions of stimulus dollars were spent to purchase and implement the Electronic Health Records mandate across the country, we now know that the outcomes have been disappointing. There have been numerous published opinions, challenges, lengthy and costly implementation processes, and failures to achieve the desired outcomes of this mandate. This is not surprising.

The purchase and implementation of the EHR was *not* seen as a major polarity that needed to be leveraged. Few began the implementation journey realizing they were taking on a major polarity, that is, the Technology (EHR) Platform and Practice Platform polarity. There was desire for the greater purpose to transform healthcare, but for many leaders, they were unaware that both poles must be supported in order to reach the greater purpose. The common approach was to see the mandate to implement the EHR as a solution to a problem.

A Clinical Scenario:

A workshop was scheduled with the leaders of a large healthcare system to address approaches to improve clinical outcomes. The meeting got off to a brisk start. The chief executive welcomed everyone and then shared his concerns that they had spent over 300 million dollars on the purchase and implementation of the EHR without any clear positive clinical outcomes. He asked the group, "What is wrong with this picture, and what are you as leaders going to do about it?"

The room filled with a tense silence. The leader of the workshop asked him, "When you signed the multimillion dollar contract for the EHR, what was your goal and your commitment? Did you commit to automate as quickly as possible and meet the meaningful-use deadlines so they could receive financial support? Or did you commit to transform the culture and practice at the point of care to improve safety and quality using technology?"

The CEO didn't miss a beat. He immediately began to explain that he knew exactly why he made the decision to automate as quickly as possible. In defense of his thinking, he explained that at the time, he believed that "anything that cost that amount of money should take care of any problems related to practice."

The call to automate the EHR is very different from the call to transform cultures and practices using technology. Leaders *must* see the whole of reality: you need the technology *and* you need to improve safety and improve quality of practice *at the same time*.

Lessons Learned

The EHR mandate caused a flurry of activity and national focus on the technology platform. As this chapter's clinical scenario shows, leaders knew
is that it matters where you get healthcare and it matters who gives the care. Over the past 30 years, that the implementation of technology would open up many possibilities and opportunities to improve practices. The hope was that the right technology would offer healthcare the same kind of exponential growth seen in the technology world to be experienced in the practice world.

That perspective is easy to understand when one takes a look at the technology world. As we all know, human evolution took place slowly, but who among us has not marveled at the incremental speed at which new technologies are being developed and applied in more ways than we can count? We need to look no further than the history of the telephone. What can we learn about exponential growth in the technology world that gives insight into achieving exponential growth in the practice field?

Exponential growth is based on the principles of science and requires a consistent, working platform or foundation. The revolution of the phone started with a working platform (the best for the time). Using the phone as an example for exponential growth, we know the growth was possible because there was a consistent working platform based on standards and principles. Once that was achieved, the next step was to improve that platform in an ongoing manner. We have all observed that exponential growth.

The practice platform, on the other hand, is not solid or consistent. There is major *variability* in the delivery of care as evidenced by errors, adverse events, omission, commission, duplication, repetition, concern for safety, quality, and cost-effectiveness. The reality the focus of the CPMRC International Consortium was to delineate the fundamental elements/components of a strong practice platform. They are

- shared purpose and clarity about the things that matter most to the healthcare mission;
- strong abilities to engage in dialogue and meaningful conversation;
- partnership (healthy healing) relationships;
- a clear understanding of each person's unique scope of practice/service;

- competency in their scope of practice/service responsibilities;
- integrated competency that can stop duplication and repetition;
- a partnership structure in daily working environments to support interprofessional networking within and across the continuum of care;
- the latest evidence-based tools and information at their fingertips that are necessary for the development of an individualized, interprofessional, integrated plan of care;
- integrated documentation that accurately reflects the recipient of care's story, plan, progress, and outcomes across the continuum of care;
- a professional exchange process/handoff that ensures the continuation of safe, quality care across the continuum.

Members of the CPMRC International Consortium representing over 400 health-care organizations around the country found that there was little consistency on the major elements/components of the practice platform. Equally important, the consortium noted that the fundamental work necessary to achieve consistency in the practice platform has not been done in most organizations. A survey was prepared to collect relevant information from thousands of clinicians. Results confirmed that there was little consistency in the strength of the practice components. The CPMRC published feedback from 6,358 interprofessional providers from multiple disciplines, including clinicians, managers, administrators, and educators from 100 clinical settings on the strength of the components taken over a six-year period (2006–2011).

Following a description of the practice components, the survey participants evaluated how strong and consistent the fundamental element was in their practice world, using the 1–5 numerical scale as shown below:

1. Describes the element as rarely strong or consistent
2. Describes the element as strong and consistent approximately 25% of the time
3. Describes the element as being strong and consistent 50% of the time
4. Describes the element as being strong and consistent 75% of the time
5. Describes the fundamental element as almost always strong and consistent

The graphic on the following page shows that each of the fundamental practice elements are variable. Without each element being strong and consistent there will be *no* way to achieve exponential growth of the practice platform. Without the practice platform being strong, the ability to reach the greater purpose of the Technology (EHR) Platform and Practice Platform polarity will not be achieved. Polarities are 100% predictable. It is this point that explains why many efforts to implement the EHR have not achieved the desired clinical outcomes.

We have lived so long with the variability of the practice platform that we have come to accept it as normal. Action steps must be taken to strengthen this pole.

Fundamental Elements
Feedback – Over 6,358 participants

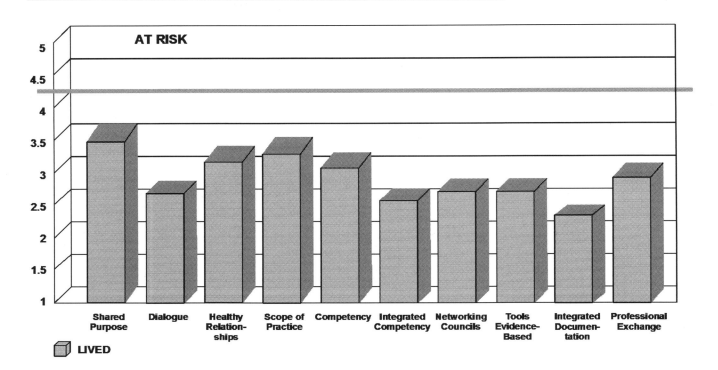

Fundamental Elements
Feedback – Over 6,358 participants

History of the Polarity

The Technology (EHR) and Practice Platform polarity map provides insights into leveraging the polarity and reaching the greater purpose: **transformation at the point of care**. If leaders had been aware that the Electronic Health Record mandate presented a major inherent polarity, the approaches, action steps, and direction of many organizations would have been very different. The process of implementation would have begun by first making sure everyone involved was clear about how the technology would function and integrate with the major practice values that needed to be maintained, strengthened, or completely changed. Polarity Thinking requires us to be clear and precise regarding the fundamental elements of the technology platform and the practice platform.

Completed Map for the Technology (EHR) Platform and Practice Platform Polarity

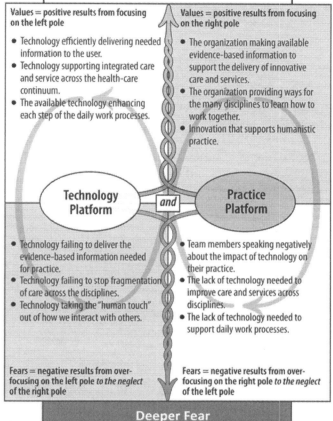

Greater Purpose Statement (GPS)
Transformation at the Point of Care
Why leverage this polarity?

Action Steps (left)
How will we gain or maintain the positive results from focusing on this left pole? What? Who? By when? Measures?

A. Clarify the benefits and limitations of the tools.
B. Ensure that users understand and can modify the design, purpose, and functionality of the technology tool.
C. Provide time for users to learn the technology tool properly.
D. Create and sustain a strong partnership with the practice team.

Values = positive results from focusing on the left pole

- Technology efficiently delivering needed information to the user.
- Technology supporting integrated care and service across the health-care continuum.
- The available technology enhancing each step of the daily work processes.

Values = positive results from focusing on the right pole

- The organization making available evidence-based information to support the delivery of innovative care and services.
- The organization providing ways for the many disciplines to learn how to work together.
- Innovation that supports humanistic practice.

Action Steps (right)
How will we gain or maintain the positive results from focusing on this right pole? What? Who? By when? Measures?

A. Practice experts commit to bring evidence-based content that supports scope of practice for interdisciplinary team.
B. Create and support time for inter-disciplinary team to do transformation work needed to integrate evidence-based professional practice by using technology.
C. Provide process that assures what matters most to both those who give and receive care is embedded into technology.
D. Create and sustain a strong partnership with technology team.
E. Assess the reality of practice at the point of care. Do a gap analysis to adequately determine how to bridge the gap and transform practice.

Technology Platform *and* **Practice Platform**

- Technology failing to deliver the evidence-based information needed for practice.
- Technology failing to stop fragmentation of care across the disciplines.
- Technology taking the "human touch" out of how we interact with others.

- Team members speaking negatively about the impact of technology on their practice.
- The lack of technology needed to improve care and services across disciplines.
- The lack of technology needed to support daily work processes.

Early Warnings (left)
Measurable indicators (things you can count) that will let you know that you are getting into the downside of this left pole.

A. Timelines for "activation" are all about technology, not practice transformation.
B. Heavy modification or deconstruction of evidence-based content integration.
C. No money to support proper education of staff for practice changes, only for use of technology.

Early Warnings (right)
Measurable indicators (things you can count) that will let you know that you are getting into the downside of this right pole.

A. Negative comments that technology is not good for clinicians or patients.
B. Users demand that technology not change what is known and familiar; i.e., documentation practices.
C. Comments about the fear that technology will dehumanize care and dictate practice.

Fears = negative results from over-focusing on the left pole *to the neglect of the right pole*

Fears = negative results from over-focusing on the right pole *to the neglect of the left pole*

Deeper Fear
Unable to Transform Practice at Point of Care
Loss of Greater Purpose

Reflections on the Technology (EHR) Platform and Practice Platform Polarity

The completed map above shows some of the desired outcomes when the technology platform is strong. The technology platform is capable of efficiently delivering needed evidence-based information to the fingertips of the users. It should encompass standardization and integration of information; increase access, retrieval, and delivery of patient information across the care continuum; and enhance each step of the interprofessional user's daily thought and work processes. Combined with the positive outcomes of the practice platform, it will lead to the desired greater purpose of *transformation at the point of care.*

The upsides of the Practice pole. When the Practice pole is strong, the information delivered to the user is evidence based and supports innovative care. There is a structure to bring interprofessional teams together to carry out their work and stop duplication and repetition of care. There is innovation that supports humanistic practice, including knowing the person's story (body, mind, and spirit), and care driven by using interprofessional, individualized plans of care across the continuum.

Knowing the desired outcomes is not enough. Clear action steps designed to keep each pole strong are necessary.

If the point of introducing new technologies is to increase efficiency, accessibility, and accountability, then everything must be done to involve those who have to use the new system *before and during implementation*. Those staff members at the point of care must be allowed to explain what they will need before a system is selected. However, feedback from healthcare management professionals indicates that this is seldom done, despite the fact that the functionality of the technology platform will markedly influence the usability of that tool by all users. Therefore, it is essential to know how each component of the product affects each component of the desired *practice* platform for practitioners. Everyone in the organization must be clear about the strength of the fundamental elements of the practice platform.

Leveraging the polarity. Knowing reality is critical in managing polarities. Knowing the status of the practice platform is essential yet often this step was neglected. The major focus was on the new technology purchased. If there is not clarity on the present and desired consistency of the Practice pole, the ability to determine the best technology tool will be less effective. The most common approach to purchase the Electronic Health Record was clarifying the benefits and limitation of the technology tool as presented by the vendor. Once purchased, the users were provided with overviews on the nature and functionality of the technology. The benefits and value of the technology *as related to the essence of the users' professional practice was often not even part of the mandatory preparation.*

The major focus was on strengthening the Technology pole, but the nature of the work to raise the consistency of the practice platform to the highest standards was often not considered. There were many early warnings about over-focusing on Technology, especially evident in the timelines for *activation* that were built around technology implementation instead of around supporting changes in practice. Many leaders report that funding was inadequate for staff training related to practice changes. The focus on technology often led to a failure to integrate evidence-based content that was needed to improve and advance practice.

The CPMRC International Consortium focused on actions steps necessary to strengthen the practice platform. The first step was to assess the strength of the fundamental elements of the practice platform and delineate the work necessary to bridge the gap between reality and the desired future. Accountability was stressed. Every member of the teams had to help develop and carry out action steps to strengthen the clinicians' use of evidence-based content for individual and interprofessionally integrated practices. The action steps called for the staff members in clinical settings to set aside time and resources so the interdisciplinary teams could do transformation work at the point of care while simultaneously developing and sustaining partnering relationships in order to stop duplication, repetition, errors, and unintended consequences.

Taking time to remain human and have a shared purpose for the interprofessional team is at the core of a practice platform. The action steps are focused on what matters most. They emphasize the need to have support for the delivery of professional scope of practice/service, knowing each patient's story and creating an individualized plan of care using the latest evidence and an education and professional exchange process for the continuum of care. In addition, a strong partnership with the technology team needs to be established.

Some clinicians were very resistant to the Technology pole because the Practice pole was being neglected. There was a great fear that the technology would dehumanize their practice and interfere with their work flow and the quality of care. Many believed that all that mattered were the timelines given by technology leaders for implementation. There was little understanding that together the Technology (EHR) Platform and Practice Platform polarity would transform practice to a higher level if done properly. There also was not a clear understanding of the depth of change needed in their daily practice.

The lack of understanding that the technology (EHR) platform and the practice platform are interdependent explains why so many EHR implementations were unable to achieve sustainable improvement in clinical outcomes and cost containment.

The EHR mandate is a timely example of just how useful Polarity Thinking is for the healthcare industry. If we don't ask whether the mandate is simply a problem to be solved or part of a polarity that must be managed (or both), we will continue to waste time and resources. Polarity Thinking explains why exponential growth has not been able to be achieved in healthcare at the point of care in the same way technology has seen exponential growth.

Chapter 12

Lessons Learned from Well-Managed Polarities

This facility has been the recipient of many awards. The effort to achieve recognition and awards such as the Magnet Recognition and the Malcolm Baldridge awards is hard work. Our leadership team has presented at multiple conferences and large organizations about the team's success and what they did to make it happen. One conference participant stood up and asked our team a question we had not anticipated. "We're already doing much of what you have done, but we didn't get the same results. What are you doing to sustain your outcomes?" Getting the award is one thing. Sustaining the outcomes is another.

Parker Palmer—activist, visionary, nationally respected educator, and author—recognized the importance of reaching a tipping point beyond which everything changes. "The starting point of a movement," he wrote, "though silent and barely visible, can be described with some precision. It happens when isolated individuals who suffer from a situation that needs changing decide to live 'divided no more.'" He maintains that there is no punishment worse than the one we inflict on ourselves by living a divided life. The gift of polarities is that it helps you see that you no longer have to live a life divided.

Polarity Thinking helps individuals and groups understand that many of our most difficult dilemmas are not simple problems that can be addressed with *either/or* thinking. It helps teach us that choosing one alternative over the other is not always the answer. Most of us have been in positions where we were asked to pick one pole or the other: "*Either* you are on this train with our team and support this cost-containment effort, *or* we leave without you." If you have a "problem" mindset, it is one or the other, and you will feel forced to choose.

We have all felt divided and untrue to our own knowing when we can see advantages on both sides. So how *can* we live divided no more?

We choose both and leverage their respective strengths equally.

The Process for Leveraging Polarities

There is a process for leveraging polarities well. In this chapter, we will use points made earlier in the book to describe how to do it.

1. **Define the difficulty.** Determine if the dilemma represents a problem to be solved, a polarity to be managed, or both. This diagnosis is critical.

   - Review with the team the difference between problems that need to be solved and interdependent pairs of values that must be leveraged.

   - Start by discussing the characteristics of a problem to solve and asking: *Is there one right answer?* Okay. Then this can be solved.

   - Review with the team the characteristics of a polarity. A polarity has two or more values that are equally important.

- Review the following criteria that must be present for a polarity to exist:
  — There are two or more necessary upsides.
  — Over-focusing on one pole will undermine the greater purpose.
  — It is an ongoing difficulty, such as breathing.
  — It has alternatives that need each other over time.

2. **Include key stakeholders.** Key stakeholders are needed to help create accurate map content, which assures an understanding of the upsides for each of the interdependent values. Key stakeholders will resist a process that does not include their point of view, but they will be great resources for polarities that do include their point of view. The content of the maps used in this book were based on the expertise of hundreds of clinicians in multiple settings across the continent. They reflect common desires and concerns.

   - It is important that the information used in this process is customized for each setting.
   - Decide who will lead the effort to support both poles.
   - Decide who will carry out the action steps.
   - Make sure to involve those people who are affected on a regular basis by the Greater Purpose and the Greater Fear/Concern. Make sure their voices are heard.

3. **Build the polarity map.** Fill in the components of the map, including the neutral names for each pole, the upside and downside for each pole, and the greater purpose and deeper fear/concern. The greater purpose is the reason why efforts should be made to reach both upsides. Neither pole can reach the greater purpose alone, so be sure that the group agrees on each component of the map. It must honor their values and fears.

4. **Determine the action steps necessary to support each pole.** Identify the realities related to each of the listed desired outcomes. The desired outcomes provide direction for the nature of the work. The action steps are necessary to achieve each outcome. What will become apparent as you decide on the action steps for one pole is that you will notice an action step may also support the other pole. That is a high-leveraged action that might need to be considered a priority for action.

5. **Create the early warnings.** It is important to know if and when one pole is being focused on to the neglect of the other pole. The early warnings help us stay vigilant and remind us that this is not a problem to be solved. We still must pay attention to both poles. It is easy to focus on the pole that is most valued and supported either by history, habit, or power over realities. Resist that impulse.

6. **Make sure everyone on board understands how polarities work.** The previous chapters have explained how polarities work. To review, there is an ongoing oscillation of the natural tension/energy between the poles that looks like an infinity loop. What drives that oscillation is the anticipation or experience of the downside of one pole, combined with the attraction to the upside of the other pole. The whole purpose is to reach the greater purpose. If you over-focus on one pole, over time you reach the limits of that pole. This makes the other pole increasingly attractive. There are virtuous and vicious cycles that can occur because of the natural tension that exists between each pole. When there is synergy between the two poles, and actions are taken to support each pole, the greater purpose is achieved and sustained through this virtuous cycle. When one pole is focused on at the neglect of the other, there is a downward or vicious spiral to the deeper fear/concern.

   A polarity pair represents two points of view. Each pole represents a point of view that is composed of the valued upside and the fear of the downside of the opposite pole. A person strongly supportive of change has a fear that the stability pole will cause stagnation.

Often the downside of the opposite pole is seen as a problem and the preferred pole value is seen as a solution. However, within a polarity there is no problem or solution—there is only an interdependent relationship between opposites that needs to be managed or leveraged.

The complete map is not about a solution, but rather about an ongoing process of leveraging and achieving a healthy balance toward the greater purpose. It requires *vigilance*.

7. **Establish a process to evaluate how well the polarities are being managed.** This is all about outcomes. Leaders in healthcare have been mandated to demonstrate outcomes. Quality outcomes and methods to manage and report them are not new to anyone dealing with operations, finance, credentialing, provider contracts, or customer impact. Measures based on interdependent pairs have not been part of evaluation processes because polarities are not a part of the established formats today. However, once a person becomes aware of polarities, it is natural to ask, "How can we tell if we are leveraging or managing the identified polarities?" The next chapter will review a new tool that addresses this issue.

Chapter 13

Polarities and the Organization: How Well Are You Managing Yours?

"How wonderful that we have met with a paradox! Now we have some hope of making progress."

— Neils Bohr, physicist

Today's healthcare leaders are expected to demonstrate outcomes of their efforts to maintain or improve healthcare according to expectations and demands. Innovation plays a huge part in our efforts to meet leaders' expectations and compete. At the roots of innovation we find a world of new ideas and ways of thinking. The polarity approach takes these seemingly disparate views and synchronizes them to reach a goal that would not be possible without collaborative leveraging. Thinking in terms of *both/and* and *either/ or* might take some getting used to, but once you have a basic understanding, you can apply the same principles to all polarities. We are surrounded with dilemmas and paradoxes, but once we accept the realities of the culture and the practice, we can use the tools to manage the leveraging process with vigilance.

The metrics that address problem-solving success are insufficient for addressing whether an organization is managing or leveraging polarities well. Barry Johnson, who developed the Polarity Thinking approach, was determined to find a process that would provide real-time diagnostic information about the effectiveness of efforts being made to strengthen each pole in order to reach the greater purpose or desired goals.

The tool he developed to operationalize the principles and structure of Polarity Thinking is referred to as the Polarity Approach to Continuity and Transformation (PACT). A Web-based survey tool was developed in partnership with Johnson that provides specific diagnostic and remediation information about how well the healthcare polarities are being leveraged in a user-friendly format and with a quick turnaround. The tool gives real-time information about the outcomes of efforts to support each pole, as well as remediation information used for future action steps. The Polarity Assessment for Healthcare (PAH) serves as a framework consisting of a polarity map template based on the components and principles of Polarity Thinking. The PAH shows high validity and reliability.

What information do we need so that we know how well we are managing polarities? The answer to this question sits in the understanding of the principles of polarities and a completed map. The desired positive outcomes and negative outcomes are listed on the map. The reporting process should give feedback about the reality related to each statement and insights into the impact of the action steps necessary to support the positive statements and prevent the negative statements. The information provides answers to such questions as

Why do we do so well at all the projects we initiate in the organization, but seem unable to sustain the changes over time?

How do we provide evidence-based consistent care, while meeting the individual needs of the patient and families?

How do we automate without dehumanizing the care we give to patients and families?

The purpose of the tool is to provide information that shows how well the overall polarity is being managed. This requires metrics that reflect the reality around the positive and negative statements on the map. The tool was set up in a familiar survey format. Those people who are stakeholders for the polarities are the ones who provide feedback.

The people taking the survey do not need to know anything about polarities. They only need to use a simple survey tool with a scale to describe their daily reality related to the upside and downside behaviors or outcomes of the positive and negative quadrants.

The participants have the following choices about how often in the last six months (the timeline can be changed for each organization) the participant observed or experienced the statement behaviors in terms of outcomes (almost never, seldom, sometimes, often, or almost always). For the positive behaviors, it would be desirable if they replied either "often" or "almost always." For the negative behaviors, it would be desirable to have them respond "seldom" or "almost never."

There are points allocated and analyzed behind the scenes, with 100 points the maximum for each quadrant. A full 100 points for each positive quadrant would be "almost always" for each statement. For the negative quadrants, 100 points would be for "almost never." A well-leveraged or managed polarity overall should be between 80–100 points. The number to reflect the overall management of the polarity is achieved by finding the means for each item in the quadrant; the mean for the quadrant score; and then the overall mean for the four quadrants. Once the survey is completed by participants, a report is spontaneously generated within five minutes that shows the collective results.

The Evaluation Process

One example of what the tool can provide comes from two different organizations that used the Polarity Assessment for Healthcare. The results from site A and site B relate to how well they are leveraging the Mission and Margin polarity. Because Polarity Thinking is new in healthcare, the researchers administering the survey predicted that when the 13 common polarities at four different sites (two in Canada and two in the United States) would be evaluated that few settings would be managing them at the highest level of 80–100 points.

The results showed that the mean for all four sites ranged from 56–69 points. In our study of four organizations, the researchers also predicted that the Mission (quality of care) and Margin (cost of care) polarity would be the lowest balanced polarity because first of all Mission and Margin was not historically addressed as a polarity, and Margin was seen as a problem to be handled by management with little engagement of staff for ownership of this pole. However, the staff did have ownership for the Mission pole. Secondarily, the survey was taken during a major recession and the rising costs of healthcare were a national issue.

Results and Outcomes of Polarity Assessment Tool for Healthcare

Margin/Cost of Service AND Mission/Quality of Service

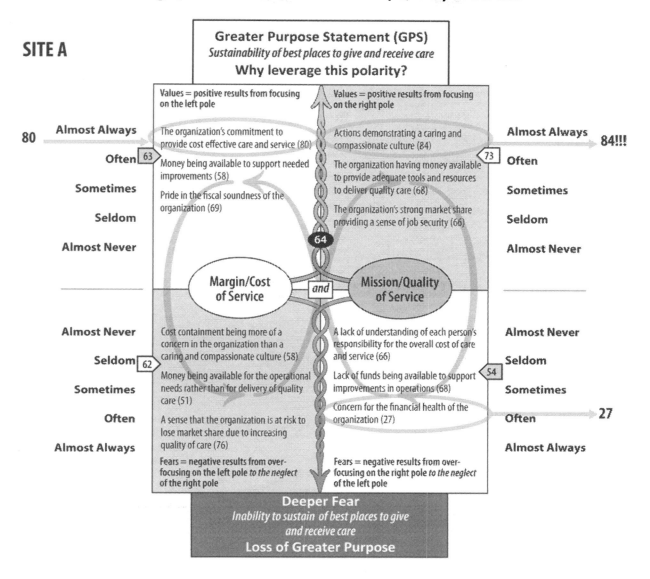

SITE A

Greater Purpose Statement (GPS)
Sustainability of best places to give and receive care
Why leverage this polarity?

Values = positive results from focusing on the left pole

Values = positive results from focusing on the right pole

80 — Almost Always

The organization's commitment to provide cost effective care and service (80)

Actions demonstrating a caring and compassionate culture (84)

Almost Always — 84!!!

Often — 63

Money being available to support needed improvements (58)

The organization having money available to provide adequate tools and resources to deliver quality care (68)

73 — Often

Sometimes

Pride in the fiscal soundness of the organization (69)

The organization's strong market share providing a sense of job security (66)

Sometimes

Seldom

Seldom

64

Almost Never

Almost Never

Margin/Cost of Service — *and* — Mission/Quality of Service

Almost Never

Cost containment being more of a concern in the organization than a caring and compassionate culture (58)

A lack of understanding of each person's responsibility for the overall cost of care and service (66)

Almost Never

Seldom — 62

Money being available for the operational needs rather than for delivery of quality care (51)

Lack of funds being available to support improvements in operations (68)

54 — Seldom

Sometimes

Sometimes

Often

A sense that the organization is at risk to lose market share due to increasing quality of care (76)

Concern for the financial health of the organization (27)

Often — 27

Almost Always

Almost Always

Fears = negative results from over-focusing on the left pole *to the neglect* of the right pole

Fears = negative results from over-focusing on the right pole *to the neglect* of the left pole

Deeper Fear
Inability to sustain of best places to give and receive care
Loss of Greater Purpose

The map above shows the results of the assessment tool for site A for the Mission and Margin polarity. Note that site A is only tapping this polarity at 64 out of 100 points (see circle in middle). This lower range came as a surprise because this organization has historically been very strong in managing many polarities. In the study, they consistently scored the highest in achieving balance for 12 out of the 13 polarities.

Notice how strong certain items in the positive quadrant are: Item (1) in Margin: "The organization's commitment to provide cost-effective care" is at 80 points, and Item (1) in Mission: "The organization's actions demonstrate a caring and compassionate culture" is at 84. These behaviors are very positive and indicate that action steps have been taken to keep both poles strong. The organization was vigilant on maintaining its mission, but also its margin. Why then is their status on this pole only 64?

An interesting thing happened. During the four-week period that the survey was taken, a major stressor appeared. For the first time in the history of this clinical setting, there were position cutbacks. Because the tool gives a real-time overview, notice how quickly this reality brought those taking the survey to evaluate the presence of the negative behaviors: "Concern for the financial health of the organization" was "often" with an average of only 27 points.

It is evident that the organization had moved into the downside of Mission and was experiencing the loss of a strong Margin. The whole quadrant is lower, but it is clear where their concerns were.

It appears that this is a recent stressor in the organization, because the other positive behaviors are still pretty good, yet the negative behavior around Concern for the Financial Health of the Organization was very high. The status of "Often" needs to be addressed and focused on. As their chief executive noted, they realized that this polarity was out of balance and that action steps needed to be taken. They had already begun to take action. The leadership met with the leaders of their partnership structure and all staff members and shifts to explain, seek input, and discuss the actions and its correlation to the Mission and Margin balance of their organization. The real-time evaluation showed the need for this action to be taken because of the strong presence of one negative behavior.

It is interesting to compare this polarity map to another site: B, which had been having Margin problems for many months before the survey was taken. It was the major focus across the setting.

Margin/Cost of Service AND Mission/Quality of Service

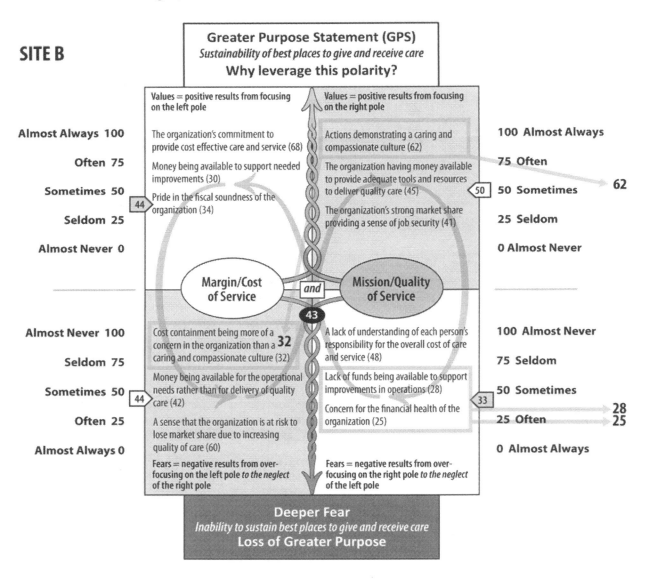

This facility is in the danger zone and is clearly not managing this polarity, because its overall number was 43 out of 100. The overall number is the mean for all four quadrants. It is low because neither pole is being leveraged or adequately supported (the mean is 44 out of 100 for Margin in the upper positive quadrant and 50 in the upper positive quadrant of the Mission pole) It is evident that the facility is in the downside of both poles and is getting negative outcomes (with a mean of 44 in the Margin pole and 33 in the Mission pole). Notice the infinity loop: The energy flow is moving into the downside of each pole.

These numbers represent real-time realities. Again, we cannot stress enough the fact that every polarity has to be managed over time, so it is important to know all the relevant history, because it often explains the numbers and the significance for each of the positive and negative statements.

Site B's History

Two years before this assessment, the team began intense work to strengthen the mission (quality of care) at the staff level. There was a strong emphasis on the mission of caring and compassion, and the tools and resources needed by staff to deliver quality care and get positive outcomes. Notice the results of the survey at this moment in time.

The efforts, which began two years ago, are still evident. The highest positive statement of the assessment was this: "Actions are demonstrating a caring and compassionate culture with a mean of 62." One might suspect that the means of the Mission pole during the year of emphasis would have all been higher, but this information was not available.

During this time of focusing on the Mission, the organization was not taking actions to strengthen the Margin side by engaging staff in knowledge and input into fiscal issues and concerns. In a problem-solving mindset, it was the managers who took care of the fiscal problems and the staff members who worked on the Mission or clinical problems. Each pole was seen as a problem to solve.

The downside of Mission was predictable and was still evident later on, with two out of three negative behaviors coming in at 25 and 28. There was often a loss of the positives of the other pole, Margin.

As the financial problems deepened, the leadership decided to solve the fiscal problem. They took several strong fiscal actions, yet paid little attention to Mission. This went on for over a year *before this survey was taken.* "No Margin, No Mission" was the mantra of the leadership. Now we see from the numbers that the organization was going into the downside of the margin pole—after all, they were focusing on this pole with great intensity for a year, and paying little attention to Mission! The result was that they were not able to raise the positive behaviors of the margin pole (a 44 mean in the upper quadrant of Margin).

Additionally, because of the neglect of the Mission pole, there was a marked increase in negative outcomes (a 44 mean in the negative column, showing the loss of the positive outcomes of the Mission pole). This is evident in the statement "Cost-containment being more of a concern in the organization than a caring and compassionate culture" (32, which is close to "often" on the scale). The vicious cycle is now in play, and those taking the survey at this time are experiencing the downsides of both poles.

A summary of what has happened. During the intense focus on Mission, which began two years before this survey, the setting was moving to the downside of Mission because people were not adequately focusing on the Margin pole. The lingering results are still evident, with two of the three downsides experienced "often" ("Concern for the financial health of the organization" sat at 25 out of 100 points, and "Lack of funds being able to support improvements in operation" fell to 28).

In a *pendulum effect,* the leaders in the organization decided to solve the fiscal problem. In the months prior to the survey, the organization was intensely focused on Margin and began to lose the previous Mission upsides, "cost-containment" being more of a concern in the organization than "a caring and compassionate culture"—it was at 32 points at this point.

The financial stress has gone on for over a year. The organization was unquestionably in the downside of Margin because leaders were only focusing on this pole for the previous months before the survey was taken. The participants from Site B believed that they were losing support for the Mission behaviors; today they are in the downside of both poles.

One thing is very important about polarities:

It doesn't matter which pole you focus on, if you neglect the other pole, you will eventually have negative outcomes and certainly fail to reach the greater purpose.

With polarities, it is essential to be vigilant and to focus on both poles *simultaneously.* When one pole is neglected, you go to the downside—but if the other pole is not strengthened, you cause a vicious cycle, and it will over time lead to the downside of both poles. You lose twice! That was what was happening in Site B. Within the evaluation tool for polarities, there is a place for each person to make a comment related to each statement. What was clear in the comments from Site B was that at that time, there were warning signs for over-focusing on Margin and a weakening of the Mission pole. Staff members were fighting for Mission, and administration was fighting for Margin. Neither will win because this is not a problem to solve. It is a polarity, and that needs to be leveraged.

The ability to differentiate problems from polarities and then diagnose, treat, and evaluate how well common polarities are being leveraged is new in healthcare. When polarities are recognized and understood, as reported by the rank-and-file of the organization through the participative process, the action steps designed to help the organizations reach common desired goals are achieved with higher ownership, less resistance, and greater speed. Equally important is having a tool that provides feedback in real time. This will save time, money, and resources.

Section Two:
Polarities for Successful Healthcare Transformation

This section presents six polarities that are particularly relevant in the process to transform the healthcare system.

Section Two

Polarities for Successful Healthcare Transformation

A. The Evidence-Based (EB) Standardized Care and Autonomous Care Polarity

"Medicine is not only a science, but also the art of letting our own individuality interact with the individuality of the patient."

— Albert Schweitzer

We discussed patient and staff safety in Chapter 10. One major polarity that impacts safety is Evidence-Based Standardized Care and Autonomous Care.

The commitment to provide evidence-based care and also make autonomous decisions to individualize care presents opportunities for conflict. Both are important realities in an efficient and compassionately run organization. No matter what the specific safety concerns are—medication errors, failure to rescue, omission or variation of care—both poles of this polarity must be addressed simultaneously. The greater purpose to create the best place to practice and receive care cannot be achieved without both values being leveraged. Once you understand the dynamic of this polarity, you will have greater insights into the recommendations coming from national organizations such as the Institute of Medicine, National Patient Safety and Quality Councils, and Joint Commission, etc.

Every day, millions of people around the world enter into a place of treatment and cure and become somebody's "patient." Safety must be a major concern of every individual. The positive outcomes of focusing on Evidence-Based Standardized Care are numerous. Organizations committed to safety/quality will have frameworks and processes in place that are evidence-based and that help the practitioners master the fundamental elements of quality care and best practices. Clear expectations, appropriate technology, and sound policies, procedures, and protocols will decrease the variations of care, which will prevent accidents and injuries, as well as errors. When this pole is strong, patients feel safe and have a sense of trust and confidence in the providers. Successful credentialing and accrediting enhances the organization's reputation.

A completed map for evidence-based standardized care and autonomous care polarities is provided on the following page.

Completed Map for Evidence-Based (EB) Standardized Care and Autonomous Care Polarity

Greater Purpose Statement (GPS)
Individualized quality care across the continuum
Why leverage this polarity?

Action Steps
How will we gain or maintain the positive results from focusing on this left pole? What? Who? By when? Measures?

A. Assure clarity on the professional, legal, financial, and credentialing standards.
B. Implement evidence-based tools and infrastructures to support standardization of care/services for all disciplines across the continuum
C. Provide opportunities to learn, evaluate, and clarify standards of care

Values = positive results from focusing on the left pole

- The team's understanding of the standards of practice that leads to safe, clinical outcomes
- Care and services being delivered according to defined standards of best practice
- The team being held accountable for the same best practice standards across the continuum of care

Values = positive results from focusing on the right pole

- Individuals having a sense of control over their practice
- The freedom of the team members to share new ideas about care that varies from standards
- Support to use professional expertise with evidence-based information to adapt practice to meet patient needs

Action Steps
How will we gain or maintain the positive results from focusing on this right pole? What? Who? By when? Measures?

A. Implement methods to measure process and outcomes of individualized care/services delivered.
B. Implement tools and resources to support critical thinking and reasoning related to professional scope.
C. Provide point of care critical tools designed to clarify patient/family values and uniqueness.
D. Provide opportunities to engage in clinical research and apply to practice.

Evidence-Based Standardized Care *and* **Autonomous Care**

Early Warnings
Measurable indicators (things you can count) that will let you know that you are getting into the downside of this left pole.

A. "All we do here is cookbook medicine."
B. "Whatever happened to professional respect?"
C. "As long as we look good, that is all that matters around here."
D. "We are victims of credentialing."
E. "I just followed the policy."
F. "Sometimes the organization and other disciplines get in the way of me delivering my full scope of practice."
G. Patient states: "Everybody does it the same, but that is not what we want to happen."
H. "People in power decide how we do it here."

- An individual's professional expertise being ignored
- The need to defend or cover up actions that vary from standardized processes
- More support for giving standardized care than for giving individualized care based on professional expertise

- Lack of understanding of standards of practice necessary to achieve safe clinical outcomes
- The care and service delivered failing to meet the defined regulations or standards
- Patient's care or service falling below standards of best practice as they move across the continuum

Early Warnings
Measurable indicators (things you can count) that will let you know that you are getting into the downside of this right pole.

A. "Everybody does their own thing around here."
B. "What you can do matters on how long you have been here."
C. Patient and families complain about inconsistency of care between providers.

Fears = negative results from over-focusing on the left pole *to the neglect* of the right pole

Fears = negative results from over-focusing on the right pole *to the neglect* of the left pole

Deeper Fear
Lack of individualized quality care across the continuum
Loss of Greater Purpose

Reflections on EB Standardized and Autonomous Care Polarity

Upsides. The desired positive outcomes of both poles are shown on the map on the previous page. Standardized care requires that each individual providing any aspect of patient care understands and works to the latest evidence-based standards and consistently delivers the care according to *best practice,* regardless of where on the continuum it is delivered. The positive outcomes of Autonomous care assure patients that the individual caring for them not only knows the most current standards, but that they also know the person's unique story—and has the autonomy to individualize their care accordingly.

Evidence-Based Standardized Care

Benefits. Keeping patients safe means that providers must follow best practice and work to evidence-based standards. When this pole is strong, individuals understand and deliver care to required standards and best practice, which will lead to safe, clinical outcomes across the continuum of care. Action steps are needed in order to make sure people not only know all the policies, procedures, routines, and patterns, but also move beyond knowing to a clarity on:

- the professional, legal, financial, and credentialing standards;

- the implementation process of evidence-based tools and frameworks to support standardization of best-practice care/services for all disciplines across the continuum;

- providing various opportunities to learn, evaluate, and clarify standards of care.

Limitations. Standardization can be rigid and stifle creativity, innovation, and enthusiasm for the work. Being safe tends to hold us back from even knowing what can be. The focus on Standardization without provider autonomy comes with rigidity, rules, protocols, and polices that will over time not only fail to make one more safe, but dehumanize those who give and those who receive care.

The early warnings will surface such as, "All we do here is cookbook medicine," "We are victims of credentialing," "I just followed the policy," and "People in power here decide how we do things."

Committed clinicians take an interest in each patient as an individual and in their hearts want to personalize what they do to meet the patient's needs. If they cannot individualize the care and cannot remove the barriers that are keeping them from meeting the unique needs of the patient, the joy and sense of pride they once took as professionals slips away. The loss of control over their practice squashes the natural desire to explore and learn ways to improve practice via research and new thinking. Clearly, action steps necessary to keep the Autonomous pole strong are missing or are being ignored.

Autonomous Care

Benefits. Autonomy/freedom in professional disciplines comes with accountability. When this pole is strong, there is pride and ownership for the professional's scope of practice, delivery, and outcomes. The caregivers establish partnerships with their patients. If they want to adapt processes in order to meet individual patients' unique needs, they have the professional expertise and evidence-based information they need. They can share new ideas about care that might vary from the norms yet might enhance the field of knowledge and raise the standards.

Action steps to strengthen the Autonomy pole include

- Implement methods to measure process and outcomes of the individualized care delivered.

- Provide the tools and resources to support critical thinking and reasoning related to each profession's scope of practice.

- Provide tools designed to clarify the patient's/family's story and values.

- Provide opportunities to engage in applied clinical research. Provider Autonomy is essential for dynamic quality care.

Limitations. When Autonomous Care is the focus and Standardization is being neglected, there will be early warnings. People will start to make comments about the inequity. "Everybody does their own thing around here." "Whoever has the power around here determines how things get done."

Patients and families will start to notice that not everybody gives the same level of direct care and that it varies from individual to individual and provider to provider. Staff members notice that there is a lot of wasted time, wasted money, and much uncertainty about what is the best care to give. When a health system puts its energy into providing Autonomous Care and virtually ignores Evidence-Based Standardization, this careless and reckless oversight is equally dangerous for those who give care as well as those who receive care.

In such circumstances, there are not likely to be structures and processes in place to offset the human weaknesses that are so common when we are expected to meet increased work demands and unexpected crises. There are no reminders or alerts built in to the daily structures and processes that help prevent errors, and there is no measure in place to **prevent** repetition, duplication, and omission. Gradually, there will be negative behaviors and outcomes; workers will pay less and less attention to standards and best practices that are designed to achieve safe clinical outcomes, and the quality of care will decline and fall short of even the minimum standards.

We instinctively know the value of concern or fear: it is an alert. It is similar to the early warnings that help us notice we are over-focusing on one pole to the neglect of the other value. It is a reminder that the action steps are not being kept in front of us. In the Standardized Care and Autonomous Care polarity, it is more natural to keep the Standardization pole in front of us because of the world situation, media coverage of hospital safety, credentialing, and the power of third-party reimbursement.

The principle to be aware of relates to the dominant-pole phenomenon: everyone else lives in the downside of the dominant pole and those who favor it are blind to its downside. The evidence of that principle has been true in this polarity. Thousands of clinicians lived in the downside of committee mandates and had to put up with new forms and processes that did not work.

We also know the paralysis fear can cause. The polarity map makes truths or values, especially those we are personally most comfortable with, so visible that others cannot deny them. It also makes visible the fears we hold around opposite or different values than our own, and in such a way, the truth and importance of the fears cannot be denied. Polarities teach us the importance and impact of fear. The principles of polarity help us to understand that often behind what we value intensely is a fear of losing that value. This fear shows up as the downside of another equally important value. *The most common fear around Standardization was that professional critical decision making would be replaced by "cookbook care" or organizational demands.*

What the polarity map makes clear is that often the action steps necessary to reach the greater purpose for safe quality care are not quick fixes and often require major tools, resources, and infrastructure changes. For example, historically the strength of healthcare organizations was that they could develop the policies and procedures. However, evidence-based tools to support the scope of practice for various interdisciplinary teams are often not available. This major intervention is in the limelight today.

Polarity Thinking appreciates the wisdom in our fears of a lost value and eliminates the paralysis of fear by leveraging the infinity loop to make sure that those legitimate fears do not become reality. So to remain safe (safety is a basic human need), we must understand polarity. Polarity Thinking honors our fears but helps us learn how to avoid being controlled by them. Everyone has fears/concerns. That truth is never going away, but Polarity Thinking teaches us a way to live securely in the face of those fears. The outcomes of leveraging the Standardized Care and Autonomous Care polarity will have an influence on how people feel. The recipient and provider will both feel safer.

Another critical polarity faced by all organizations concerned about safety is Routine Task and Scope of Practice.

B. The Routine Task and Scope of Practice Polarity

"Everyone has been made for some particular work, and the desire for that work has been put in his or her heart."

— Rumi

Introduction

This polarity plays a fundamental role in achieving safety, because it is all about what happens at the point of care. The point of care, which determines the outcomes that are so important to quality care, relates to the actual services given to the person receiving care. It is composed of the Routine Task pole and the Scope of Practice pole, as well as the specific professional accountabilities of each person providing direct care. This polarity has an important history.

History of Unipolar Focus

It is helpful to understand how the Task pole became dominant in healthcare for so many years, and how important it is for safety. Nursing in an acute care setting will be used as an example. Traditionally, when a nurse started practice in the hospital, the care was often built around doctor's orders. Nurses were accountable for providing the basic hands-on care, such as bathing, feeding, activity, and environmental factors that support healing. The major focus in the hospital was on carrying out the doctor's orders related to the medical diagnosis and treatment process, along with the hospital's routine tasks, protocols, and procedures. Orientation for new nurses was about making sure the nurses knew the usual treatments and checking them off on each one. There were mandatory in-services where you were checked-off on the use of equipment and demonstrated an understanding of new policies, procedures, and treatments ordered by physicians and hospital standards. The action steps to keep the Task pole strong were well defined and supported.

Within the Task pole, one's credibility was built on how fast you could do the tasks, whether or not you carried out all the orders during your shift, whether you left anything undone that the nurses on the next shift would have to do, and whether you finished your shift on time. These accountability measures led to the institutionalization of nursing practice. The routines of the day dictated practice: it began with a designated amount of time to get a report at the beginning of the shift about the patient's diagnosis and physiological status, and what orders were written or needed to be completed on your shift. At the end of the shift, there was a "reporting-off" within a designated time and a standard pattern of information exchange. There didn't seem to be enough time in a normal day to get it all done, and the need for additional help was a common call.

Under these conditions, certain behaviors insidiously emerged, such as the staff referring to patients by their diagnosis and room numbers, resulting in communication like this:

- "I am caring for the heart in 202."
- "I need help with the kidney in room 203."
- "Let me give you a report on the lung in 204."

Reports were full of numbers:

- "The BP is 150/90, pulse running between 90–100, respiration's 22, weight is 204#, and there are 3 IVs, one at 20, one at 30, and one at 100 cc."

- "The person has received a total of 1100 cc on this shift, his output is 500 cc urine, 100 from chest tube and 200 from NG...The 24-hour intake is positive by 500 cc."

Then there would be hemodynamic monitoring numbers, lab numbers, medications given, number of treatments done, etc. The patterns and routines became robotic, and soon you could feel the dehumanization in the air.

Ironically, Florence Nightingale warned us 150 years ago about over-focusing on the Task pole. She said, "This hospital is so busy, in such a hurry that we are falling into bad habits before we are aware." She realized that the other pole, professional nursing, was being lost. It was rare to have conversations around the professional scope of practice. Often scope was not discussed as a part of the expectations or part of the ongoing education or evaluation of performance. This nursing scenario was similar to all other interprofessional practitioners giving care at the bedside.

Completed Map for Routine Tasks and Scope of Practice Polarity

Greater Purpose Statement (GPS)
Complete processes of care/service
Why leverage this polarity?

Action Steps
How will we gain or maintain the positive results from focusing on this left pole? What? Who? By when? Measures?

A. Update and inform on policies and procedures related to fundamental (routine tasks) elements of care.
B. Provide opportunities to learn and evaluate the policies and procedures.
C. Routinely provide reviews of policy and procedures and performance.

Values = positive results from focusing on the left pole

- There is efficient delivery of routine tasks of care and services.
- Routine tasks of care and services are being delivered in a competent manner.
- Policies and procedures are followed during the delivery of routine tasks of care and service.

Values = positive results from focusing on the right pole

- Team members understand their accountabilities for their professional scope of practice.
- Team members competently deliver care based on their scope of practice.
- The team says that caring for the whole person is an important part of their scope of practice.

Action Steps
How will we gain or maintain the positive results from focusing on this right pole? What? Who? By when? Measures?

A. Provide disciplines time to delineate and dialogue about their scope of practice.
B. Provide resources and evidence-based tools to support the delivery of each element of each discipline's scope of practice.
C. Assure that continuing education supports the scope of practice.
D. Provide the educational support to learn how tools and resources support the individual and integrated scope of practice.

Routine Task Care *and* **Scope of Practice Care**

Early Warnings
Measurable indicators (things you can count) that will let you know that you are getting into the downside of this left pole.

A. "The only thing that matters around here is how much you do and how fast you can do it."
B. Professional exchange report is about tasks ordered and what was done or not done.
C. Mandatory education classes only evaluate knowledge and competency in policies and procedures.

- Team members are unable to tell the difference between scope of practice and routine tasks of care.
- There is a greater focus on accomplishing tasks rather than the delivery of scope of practice.
- The strong focus on tasks is interfering with the delivery of whole person care and services.

- There is inefficient delivery of routine tasks of care and service.
- There is a failure to competently perform routine tasks of care.
- There is a failure to follow policies and procedures in the delivery of routine tasks.

Early Warnings
Measurable indicators (things you can count) that will let you know that you are getting into the downside of this right pole.

A. There are patient complaints about tasks such as mouth care, baths, and linen changes not being done.
B. "Nobody helps get the basics done around here."
C. "Doesn't anyone know how things are usually done around here?"

Fears = negative results from over-focusing on the left pole *to the neglect* of the right pole

Fears = negative results from over-focusing on the right pole *to the neglect* of the left pole

Deeper Fear
Incomplete processes of care/service
Loss of Greater Purpose

Reflections on the Routine Task and Scope of Practice Polarity

Upsides. The positive outcomes when both poles are strong are evident in the map above. In this fast-paced world, it is important that the tasks and basic routines of care be provided in an efficient manner. All those caring for the patient when both poles are strong will be competent and will consistently carry out doctor's orders, treatments, policies and procedures. The positive outcomes of the Scope of Practice pole assure colleagues that clinicians in each discipline and/or job role are clear about their unique accountabilities within their professional scope of practice/services; use critical thinking skills to competently deliver their scope; and carry it out in the context of whole-person care—body, mind, and spirit.

Benefits. The importance of the Routine Task Pole is obvious. There is efficient, effective, and consistent delivery of basic routine tasks of care in a competent manner following the policies, protocol, procedures, and basic doctor's orders. The action steps to support the Task pole have been strong historically. Orientation, ongoing education, and performance evaluations focus on knowing and demonstrating skills related to the policies and procedures, protocols, and basic doctor orders. There are multiple opportunities to review, learn, and be evaluated on the policies and procedures.

However, when the Task pole is focused on to the neglect of the Scope of Practice pole, the early warnings will appear. There will be comments such as, "The only thing that matters around here is how much you do and how fast you can do it," "All we have time for around here is getting the tasks done," and "The only thing that matters in reports is what tasks are done or not done and whether there are any new orders." Mandatory education classes only evaluate knowledge and competency in policies and procedures, and treatment protocols.

Limitations. The downside of the Task pole produces negative quadrant outcomes such as team members being unable to articulate the difference between Scope of Practice and Routine Tasks of care. There is greater focus on accomplishing tasks, rather than on the delivery of Scope of Practice, and the strong focus on Tasks interferes with the delivery of whole person care and service. When the focus is on Tasks to the neglect of Scope of Practice, there is great danger for the person receiving care. The Scope of Practice is much more than Tasks and requires very different action steps to support it. This fact becomes apparent when the Scope of Practice is understood.

Overview of Scope of Practice Pole

The Scope of Practice pole is less understood, yet is critical to the safety and quality of care for every person. When scope is strong, each member of the team understands his/her responsibilities and competently delivers whole-person care based on his/her professional scope of practice. The importance of that statement is only evident when one is clear on what scope of practice means.

Nursing's scope will be used as an example, since it is the largest point-of-care provider. The scope of practice holds each nurse accountable to critical thinking associated with the services of their profession. For example, the first accountability of a nurse's license involves the nurse needing a doctor's order to give an antibiotic to a patient. However, the nurse does not give it just because it was ordered. This constitutes negligence, according to his/her license, and the nurse could be liable for suit. Before the nurse gives the antibiotic, he/she must check to see if the person is allergic, and check to see if a culture or sensitivity test was done. If the person is resistant or allergic, the nurse calls to get the order changed. In addition, the nurse must know the reason for giving the medication, the proper dose, and its impact on the other systems of the body and other medications, as well as the potential side effects associated with the medicine. Nurses are the only continuous 24-hour hands-on caregivers, and if they do not know the side effects, the person is at risk. That is just one component of their practice. The responses or actions of the nurse to a written order relate to the scope of practice, and those responses are often not ordered by a physician, but are a responsibility under their license.

The second accountability is to assess, monitor, detect, and prevent any complications the patient is at risk for because of his/her present diagnosis or situation. Often the patient is at risk for multiple complications. For example, if a person has a spinal-cord injury, he/she is at risk for 16 common complications. This requires in-depth knowledge and understanding. The nurse needs to know the signs and symptoms of each complication, take actions to prevent such complications, and if they occur, get medical follow-up. These preventive actions are often not ordered by the physician, but are the nurse's professional responsibility.

The third accountability within one's nursing license is that he/she must also diagnose and treat the human response to the overall situation the patient is experiencing. Common human responses are anxiety, fear, grief, and post-trauma response. This commitment is to care for the whole person and intervene as needed. It requires key expertise and wisdom to carry out this component of the nurse's scope of practice.

This brief overview of the nursing's scope of practice demonstrates the complexity and importance of this pole. The same complexity would be evident no matter what interprofessional Scope we reviewed. The Scope pole needs strong support. If one's practice is only filled with doing the tasks and not also the care and critical thinking associated with the professional scope of practice, those who give and receive care are at risk. There are no quick fixes to address this polarity. Without focus on the Scope and support for this pole, there will be **variability of the delivery of professional services.** It is obvious that quality cannot be achieved under such circumstances.

Action steps to support the Scope pole are often weak in many clinical settings. The organization needs to give people in the diverse disciplines time to delineate and dialogue about their scope of practice; provide resources and evidence-based tools to support the delivery of each element of each discipline's scope of practice; make sure that continued education supports the scope of practice; provide the educational support to learn how to use the tools and resources; and make sure the expectations of Scope become a performance norm. With these action steps, the positive behaviors and outcomes of this pole will be achieved: Each team member will understand the responsibilities for their professional scope of practice, and each team member will consistently deliver care accordingly and within a whole-person context.

Limitations. There are early warnings when there is a focus on the Scope pole to the neglect of the Task pole: patients and families complain about the lack of personal care, mouth care, and baths. Treatments and medications are late. Care is not being consistently and competently carried out. Staff members make these kinds of comments: "Nobody helps get the basics done around here" and "Doesn't anybody know how things are usually done?"

Considerations. Both of these poles need to be strong in order to achieve safe, quality care. Today many providers are living in the downside of the Task pole and need help to strengthen their Scope within the present cultures. The good news is that the traditional patterns strengthened the Task pole, as evidenced by strong policies, procedures, evaluation processes, and orientation that focused on task performance. But that same depth of support for Scope and the nature of the work necessary to strengthen Scope is not strong in many organizations. When the culture does not focus on Scope and this is combined with a strong Task focus, it becomes clear that lack of clarity on scope of practice decreases overall for the professions and weakens their ability to carry it out, resulting in the "bad habits" Nightingale noted. The action steps for the Scope of Practice pole are different and require that everyone is clear about personal license, organizational structures, new tools and resources, new evaluation processes, and a culture of continuous learning.

With the many demands placed on organizations and the workloads of the caregivers, it is hard to find the time needed for people in all the disciplines to clarify their Scope. They need evidence-based tools to support each component of their scope. With knowledge doubling each year, this is an essential area of support. The need for evidence-based tools goes beyond knowing the scope of practice to the delivery of care, including the processes and documentation of the patient's story, individual plans of care, progress, and daily professional exchange reports. Without this support, patient safety cannot be achieved.

Nursing was used as an example here, but this process is true for every other discipline (i.e., physicians; respiratory therapists; dieticians; physical, occupational, and speech therapists; social workers; pharmacists; etc.). Many lessons have been learned about this polarity within the CPMRC International Consortium of over 400 rural, community, and university settings, but one lesson stands out: We must clarify, develop, and support the scope of practice for all the interprofessional disciplines.

C. The Individual Competency and Team Competency Polarity

Introduction

It is essential to stop the variability of care, and that begins with clarity on scope of practice. However, to ensure safe, quality, and cost-effective care, it is also essential to stop duplication and repetition and make sure that the care is integrated within the team caring for an individual. Accountability for individual competency is easier to accomplish and better understood than the accountability for team competency. This is a major challenge for those leading healthcare transformation. Breaking the silos within the organization across the multiple disciplines begins by first understanding the Individual Competency and Team Competency polarity.

Completed Map for Individual Competency and Team Competency Polarity

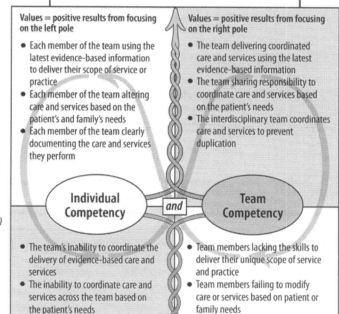

Greater Purpose Statement (GPS)
Integrated, competent care
Why leverage this polarity?

Action Steps
How will we gain or maintain the positive results from focusing on this left pole? What? Who? By when? Measures?

A. Establish processes for each person to clarify their own scope of practice.
B. Provide processes and learning opportunities to enhance critical thinking and reasoning related to each scope of practice.
C. Provide evidence-based tools to support the delivery of individual scope of practice.

Values = positive results from focusing on the left pole

- Each member of the team using the latest evidence-based information to deliver their scope of service or practice
- Each member of the team altering care and services based on the patient's and family's needs
- Each member of the team clearly documenting the care and services they perform

Values = positive results from focusing on the right pole

- The team delivering coordinated care and services using the latest evidence-based information
- The team sharing responsibility to coordinate care and services based on the patient's needs
- The interdisciplinary team coordinates care and services to prevent duplication

Action Steps
How will we gain or maintain the positive results from focusing on this right pole? What? Who? By when? Measures?

A. Provide opportunities for the team to synchronize their collective care on an ongoing basis.
B. Develop the ability of each provider to articulate their own scope, and explain the uniqueness and overlap with others' scope.
C. Assume the provision of tools and resources to enhance integration of care/services.
D. Assume the presence of the educational support needed to implement the tools and resources to integrate care.

Individual Competency *and* **Team Competency**

Early Warnings
Measurable indicators (things you can count) that will let you know that you are getting into the downside of this left pole.

A. "Physicians, nurses (or other disciplines), rule here."
B. "The only thing they care about is getting their work done."
C. "Disciplines deliver care in isolation. Everybody does their own thing."

- The team's inability to coordinate the delivery of evidence-based care and services
- The inability to coordinate care and services across the team based on the patient's needs
- Duplication of care and services across the interdisciplinary team

- Team members lacking the skills to deliver their unique scope of service and practice
- Team members failing to modify care or services based on patient or family needs
- Team members failing to clearly document the care and services they provide

Early Warnings
Measurable indicators (things you can count) that will let you know that you are getting into the downside of this right pole.

A. Complaints that some members of the team are not competent
B. Complaints that some individuals do not participate on the team
C. "No one seems to own their own accountability."
D. "It matters who takes care of you here."
E. "Some people do not document what they do or write on the plan of care."

Fears = negative results from over-focusing on the left pole *to the neglect* of the right pole

Fears = negative results from over-focusing on the right pole *to the neglect* of the left pole

Deeper Fear
Fragmented, incompetent care
Loss of Greater Purpose

Reflections on the Individual Competency and Team Competency Polarity

Upsides. The upsides of this polarity are fundamental to safe, quality, and cost-effective care as seen in the map above. The Individual Competency pole speaks to the accountability on the part of every member of the team regarding his or her scope, as well as for delivery and documentation of individualized evidence-based care. This polarity relates to the Evidence-Based Standardized and Autonomous Care and Routine Task and Scope of Practice polarities discussed in parts A and B of Section Two. Since the person receiving care is relying on a team for quality, it is imperative that every member of the team is competent and that the service he or she provides is integrated. Team competency is weaker at the point of care.

Benefits. Traditionally, the Individual Competency pole has been associated with the Task pole. As scope of practice is beginning to be recognized as an essential step to stop variability and achieve quality care, there is now greater attention paid to establishing a process to support and evaluate the Individual Competency beyond Task to include Scope. The action steps outlined in parts A and B as well as those delineated to support Individual and Team Competency are useful here.

It is natural for an individual to want to be competent and provide the best care possible. Many individuals are advancing their practice and their academic and research capabilities. This has resulted in an increase of credentialing within individual professions. More organizations are offering practice advancement/ladder programs, and more professional organizations have decided to offer certificates and recognition for advancement of knowledge and skills. *It is not that organizations have been over-focusing on the Individual Competency pole; they have been doing the necessary work of making this pole strong.* The problem is that many do not know that Individual Competency is a pole and that at the same time they need to pay attention to Team Competency to reach the greater purpose of safe, competent care. The national call to stop the errors, omission, duplication, and repetition of services that are wasting time and money represents an early warning that the Team Competency pole is being neglected. Additionally, many disciplines are delivering their care in isolation, so now we hear complaints that individuals are only focused on getting their own work done or complaints that other disciplines are interfering with their ability to deliver their care.

Team Competency. The national call is for team integration. The professions are responding, but not within a Polarity Thinking mindset. There is one important understanding about this polarity that is being missed: Team relationships are important, but team competency is also important, and it is different: it begins with partnership skills, but then the partners across disciplines must deliver their care differently. Coordination of the delivery of care requires each discipline to know the other team member's Scope; be able to clearly articulate how they build on each other's care; create an interprofessional individualized plan of care; and then coordinate the delivery of it. It is a major change in thinking and doing. *This polarity is bringing a new accountability to each person on the team, which is being accountable for his/her own competency is not enough. They are equally accountable for Team Competency.* That cannot be done without the organization taking actions to establish a team organizational structure to support the Vertical/Horizontal/Partnership polarity that provides the basis for the teams to come together and then do the hard work to stop duplication and repetition. This means that the teams have to be brought together to dialogue and discuss how to make it happen on an ongoing basis. That is a cost factor that is often not supported. If you try to hold people accountable, you must give them the support to learn and the necessary frameworks and structures for this new way of practice. Few settings offer interprofessional evidence-based guidelines to support the team during this process, and this is but one example of what will be critical if the teams are to succeed.

Action steps for this polarity. Leadership needs to have a strong understanding of the action steps, because the outcomes are correlated to sustainable safety, quality, and cost-effectiveness. The support for the fundamental work to educate the team and provide needed resources to reach the greater purpose of integrated care takes time and money. (This polarity is also markedly correlated to the Technology Platform and Practice Platform in Chapter 11.) The technology functionality needs to support the workflow of an integrated team within their scope and process, including assessment, diagnosing, planning, implementation, and evaluation. The Electronic Technology needs to deliver evidence-based interprofessional guidelines to the team, support an integrated plan of care, and integrate documentation across the team and continuum of care.

There is much work to be done to leverage this polarity.

D. Directive Decision Making and Shared Decision Making Polarity

"Relationships are all there is."

— Margaret Wheatley

Introduction

Work plays a major role in the quality of one's life. The decisions made by each person on the team have a major impact on the work culture and clinical outcomes that surround them. This polarity is about believing in the ability of colleagues to make a difference (the reason most come into the profession). It is about inclusiveness. It is about engaging them around things that matter most in their work.

There are two types of decision making: **directive decision making** and **shared decision making.** Both are essential. Each individual committed to caring for patients in a healthcare setting will be expected to make both kinds of decisions. Making the decision is only the first step. Each person is accountable for implementing the decision, owning the consequences and evaluating the outcomes.

In the work field, the question often is, "Who makes the decisions?" In healthcare, we are faced with multiple simple and complex decisions. One important fact is that everyone is accountable for the mission of the organization, and no matter who makes the decision, it should have a positive impact on the mission. In an organization, we commit to a role, position, and profession. With that comes specific accountability for certain decisions.

The polarity map on the following page offers further insights.

The Directive Decision Making Pole

Benefits of the Directive Decision-Making pole. The positive upside of the Directive pole is that individuals at all levels are trusted to be decisive and timely according to the preferences and norms of their domain and the organization. People are very clear about who is making the decision and who is accountable for the outcomes. Decision makers are clear on their scope regarding practice/service, authority, and responsibility, and they know the ways in which their decisions will support the mission and reflect the core beliefs of the organization.

Those who favor this domain know the downsides of Shared Decision Making and fear that diverse perspectives will cause chaos and offer too many choices. Conflict will increase, and those involved will not be sure who is responsible for the process and outcomes of the decision. They are likely to fear that the shared process will take too long and possibly cause team paralysis and even disengagement of the team members. It is important for those favoring the Directive pole to be aware of the early warnings that they are over-focusing on Directive Decision Making to the neglect of the Shared Decision Making pole. The "we-they" mindset is present in the culture and more employees start making frequent comments like "No one ever listens to us around here" and there is covert as well as overt resistance to new ideas. This slows down implementation of any decision. There is resistance to ideas. Changes are made, but they do not last over time because little or no attention was paid to involving everyone in the decision-making process. "Don't they have any idea how this will affect us?"

Completed Map for Directive Decision Making and Shared Decision Making Polarity

Greater Purpose Statement (GPS)
Flexible, vibrant organization
Why leverage this polarity?

Action Steps
How will we gain or maintain the positive results from focusing on this left pole? What? Who? By when? Measures?

A. Use the Partnership Council infrastructure to communicate rationale for decisions.
B. Check for concerns around implementation of directive decisions.
C. Use dialogue and partnership skills to increase trust and relationships among the team.
D. Clearly define the decision making process and accountability.
E. Evaluate the outcomes of decisions and be willing to alter plans as necessary.
F. Admit mistakes and seek wider participation whenever possible.

Values = positive results from focusing on the left pole
- Leadership is trusted to be decisive and timely with the interests of the organization in mind.
- There is clarity on who is accountable for decisions, and a willingness to make tough decisions.
- Decision makers are clear on their scope of service, authority, and responsibility.
- Decision makers are clear on how they support the mission and core beliefs.
- Leadership provides clear goals.

Values = positive results from focusing on the right pole
- There are diverse perspectives from many individuals.
- Decisions are perceived as feasible to implement and sustainable over time.
- There is a reasonably quick implementation timeline.
- There is a collective wisdom and synergistic creativity.
- There is commitment, ownership, accountability, and responsibility to decisions.
- Outcomes are owned by all.

Action Steps
How will we gain or maintain the positive results from focusing on this right pole? What? Who? By when? Measures?

A. Use the Council as an ongoing leadership group that has built strong relationships.
B. Use established tools for decision making (e.g., consensus, polarity management, and dialogue) to explore further.
C. Involve the voices of expertise from direct providers, managers, educators, researchers, and other stakeholders.
D. Set timelines for decision making and outline the process to evaluate outcomes.
E. Assure that all participants are well informed on the topic before decision making.
F. Ask how the decision focuses on the patients.

Directive Decision Making *and* **Shared Decision Making**

Early Warnings
Measurable indicators (things you can count) that will let you know that you are getting into the downside of this left pole.

A. "No one ever listens to us around here."
B. It takes a great deal of time and energy to implement new ideas.
C. There is resistance (both overt and covert) to ideas.
D. Changes are made, but they do not last over time.
E. "Don't they have any idea how that will affect us?"
F. "We/they" mentality is present in the culture.

- Decisions are made without considering diverse perspectives.
- Implementation timelines may be lengthy due to lack of overall engagement.
- It is difficult to sustain implementation changes over time.
- People whose lives are affected by decisions are excluded from the process.

- Diverse perspectives are causing chaos and too many choices.
- Conflict among decision makers is increasing.
- There is uncertainty about who is accountable for decisions and no clear goals.
- There is "analysis paralysis" among team members.
- Members might disengage from the team.

Fears = negative results from over-focusing on the left pole *to the neglect of the right pole*

Fears = negative results from over-focusing on the right pole *to the neglect of the left pole*

Early Warnings
Measurable indicators (things you can count) that will let you know that you are getting into the downside of this right pole.

A. "It takes months to make decisions around here."
B. "We have been over this same issue again and again."
C. People are not attending Council or other staff engagement sessions.
D. There is disengagement as various meetings as people think nothing will happen.
E. "I don't know who is responsible."
F. "Our Council is just a gripe session."

Deeper Fear
Unhealthy, unbalanced organization
Loss of Greater Purpose

Benefits of the Shared Decision Making pole. There are positive upsides to the Shared Decision Making pole when many individuals are asked to share their views. Diverse perspectives generally result in better decisions that are feasible to implement. What's more, the collective wisdom and creative energy from the interactions provoke group synergy that builds commitment, ownership, accountability, and responsibility to the process and outcomes of the decisions. This enhances speed of implementation and continuous learning in real time.

Those who favor this pole know some of the downsides of the Directive pole. Too many decisions made by leaders without considering diverse perspectives will result in poor decisions and slower implementation. Additionally, they know that people who are excluded from key decisions that affect their work lives will respond in diverse ways. Feelings of frustration, resistance, defiance, anger, apathy, and hopelessness are all characteristic of cultures where the decision-making process is not shared.

Limits of Shared Decision Making. It is important that those who are more inclined to favor the Shared Decision Making pole be aware of the early warnings that they are over-focusing on Shared Decision Making to the neglect of the Directive Decision Making pole, such as these signs: "It takes months to make decisions around here." "We have been over this same issue again and again." "People are not attending Council or other staff engagement sessions." People in such work cultures are less likely to engage in meeting discussions because they think nothing will happen. "I don't know who is responsible." "Our Council is just a gripe session."

Action Steps. Both poles need to be strong. When an action step is listed for both poles, it is often a priority that needs to be acted on, no matter what. This polarity is unusual in that most of the action steps on one side also appear on the other side. This polarity will not be leveraged unless there is a horizontal or partnership council infrastructure that connects all those whose wisdom and voices are needed to make a decision or those who will be affected by a decision. There are many lessons around the planning and developing of this type of foundational structure, which will eventually become embedded throughout the organization and affect everyone, regardless of position, role, or unique responsibilities. Partnerships, Dialogue, and Polarity Thinking are a part of a healthy decision-making process because they support both poles and are key to leveraging the polarity.

This polarity is closely aligned with the Vertical and Horizontal polarity. If the Vertical pole is dominant, there likely will be a stronger focus on Directive Decision Making and an absence of any policies and processes to support Shared Decision Making. If the Horizontal pole is dominant, there will be a stronger focus on Shared Decision Making. The culture of an organization where this polarity is being leveraged is vibrant and is capable of reaching good decisions that support reaching the greater purpose.

E. The Productivity and Relationships Polarity

"There is more to life than increasing its speed."

— Mahatma Gandhi

Introduction

We are living in a fast-paced practice culture. The demands are many and the available time to do the work seems too short. The cost of healthcare has been rising every year. By 2020, it is predicted it will represent 20% of our gross domestic product. The government and payers are intensely focused on the unacceptable cost of care. The Institute of Medicine (IOM) led the way with its focus in 2001 to ensure that services are safe, effective, patient-centered, timely, efficient, and equitable. The IOM continues its lead and reported in 2012 that about 30% of health spending in 2009, or roughly $750 billion, was wasted on unnecessary services. The Institute of Healthcare Improvement (2013) has developed a framework that describes an approach to optimize health system performance called the Triple Aim. Its focus is on improving the patient experience of care (including quality and satisfaction), improving the health of population and reducing the per capita cost of healthcare. The commonwealth study (2014) reported the U.S. healthcare system is the most expensive in the world. It is no surprise that at the center of healthcare transformation is the goal to decrease the rising cost of healthcare and simultaneously improve the quality of care. One of the common patterns to address the cost issue, a situation that needs to be addressed, was to increase productivity so to improve the margin. Although many organizations are working on increasing their productivity, many did not ask, "Is productivity a problem to be solved or a polarity that must be managed or both?

Productivity is not the sole accountability of any one person but all those who will give care to the person. As stated in various places in this book: There is no one person, no one discipline, no one profession, no one setting, no one researcher or scientist, no one payer who can ensure productivity, it is every one engaged in the care of an individual. Therefore, productivity is dependent on the relationships of those on the team. Often productivity was not thought of as a polarity occurring in healthcare. The focus was on getting more efficient in the delivery of care. It was thought of as another project that needed to be taken on to solve a problem.

A Clinical Scenario:

The large walk-in clinic was not meeting its numbers, and patients were beginning to complain about their care. There was talk that if the clinic could not increase its revenue, decrease its expenses, and improve the quality of care, the clinic might have to close its doors.

The message from the larger system administration was to fix this situation starting with productivity. The manager of the unit focused on the Margin pole and improving productivity. The goal was to become more efficient in performing each step in the patient intake and outtake process. If patients could be moved in and out more quickly, more patients could be accommodated in a shorter period of time, thus increasing revenue and improving patient satisfaction. A system was set up to collect time of arrival, time to reach the treatment room, and "table time." The whole process related to increasing productivity was presented to the staff. Productivity reports were given and reviewed in an ongoing manner with emphasis on best times.

The manager was diligent and evaluated the new plan on the basis of whether or not the "in and out" process was shorter for each patient, instead of evaluating the team's work productivity and patient satisfaction. It was all about working *faster*. Within a month, the stress within the unit increased and people had started to compete to see who could admit, treat, and release patients in the shortest amount of time. People who took a little more time with their patients were blamed for slowing processes further down the line. There was no time for the team to meet and discuss where there were bottlenecks and how to refine the processes. The reports and discussions were restricted to the latest time-study results as evidence of admission and discharge productivity. Things did not improve.

Reflection on the Productivity and Relationships Polarity

Productivity Pole

Raising and improving productivity are essential for the success of walk-in clinics like this one. They need positive outcomes, and everyone needs to be clear about roles, expectations, and skills necessary to deliver care in the most efficient manner as a team. Focus needs to be on getting the job done, and people need to feel personally responsible for their performance. This will give them a sense of accomplishment. The individuals, teams, and patients will all benefit from top-quality work being done in a timely manner.

Completed Map for the Productivity and Relationships Polarity

Greater Purpose Statement (GPS)
Cost effective quality care
Why leverage this polarity?

Action Steps
How will we gain or maintain the positive results from focusing on this left pole? What? Who? By when? Measures?

A. Tools and resources necessary to deliver care in the most cost-effective and efficient manner.
B. Staff engaged in the process needed to increase efficiency in workflow.
C. Staff determine the productivity measures and evaluate the impact on desired outcomes.

Values = positive results from focusing on the left pole

- There is clarity on role and expectations.
- Each person has the skills necessary to deliver care efficiently.
- There is collective attention to get the job done by holding each other accountable for most efficient integrated performance.
- There are tangible results and measurements.
- There is a sense of accomplishment by the team.

Values = positive results from focusing on the right pole

- The team is connected by a shared purpose and meaning of the work.
- Intentional nurturing relationships and clarification of what each member needs to carry out their scope of practice and service effectively and efficiently.
- There are healthy, partnering relationships between the team and the team and the people they serve.
- There is a sense of belonging and being a part of a supportive community of care that impacts the quality of life for those who give and receive care.

Action Steps
How will we gain or maintain the positive results from focusing on this right pole? What? Who? By when? Measures?

A. An ongoing partnership infrastructure in place that brings interprofessional team together to integrate and advance care.
B. Development of dialogue, partnership, and polarity thinking skills to support team integration.

Productivity *and* **Relationships**

Early Warnings
Measurable indicators (things you can count) that will let you know that you are getting into the downside of this left pole.

A. "The only thing that matters around here is how fast you can move the patients in and out."
B. "A short 'table time' is more important than the care given to the people."

- This is a loss of purpose and meaning of work
- Lack of clarity on how to support one another
- Relationships are dehumanized between both those who give and receive care
- Loss of a sense of collective ownership and connection to the quality of care

- Lack of clarity on roles and expectations to achieve cost effective care
- Lack of skills necessary to deliver care efficiently
- Unaware of the most efficient integrated workflow
- No tangible results showing productive outcomes
- Loss of sense of accomplishments

Early Warnings
Measurable indicators (things you can count) that will let you know that you are getting into the downside of this right pole.

A. Lack of clarity or ownership for how to deliver cost effective care
B. Duplication, repetition, and increased time to deliver services

Fears = negative results from over-focusing on the left pole *to the neglect* of the right pole

Fears = negative results from over-focusing on the right pole *to the neglect* of the left pole

Deeper Fear
Costly, ineffective care
Loss of Greater Purpose

Action steps. When there is a new workflow process, the team must be given the tools and resources they need to do the work in an effective and efficient manner. Staff members need to engage with one another and agree on the processes as well as determining productivity measures that would demonstrate the desired outcomes. Individual and team responsibility would be part of the process, and success of the individuals and team would be acknowledged.

Limits of Productivity. The map clearly demonstrates that if the Productivity pole is focused on to the neglect of the Relationships pole, the unit will slip into the downside of the pole. This is what happened in this case:

> The relationships necessary to increase productivity were ignored. The individuals felt that the only thing that mattered was to get the "times down."

This somewhat mechanical approach to care led to disconnected and fragmented processes and procedures, as well as feelings of dehumanization on the part of patients and those who cared for them.

Early warnings. There were early warnings. "The only thing that matters around here is how fast you can move the patients in and out." "A short table time is more important than the care given to the people." "Everybody here, including the staff, is just a number to be reported out." "I am evaluated by the length of the table time for my patients, but others were slowing me down."

Staff frustration led to dissatisfaction on the part of the team and those receiving care. People started using more sick time, and there was staff turnover during the period of the productivity time study. If this serious issue had been seen as a polarity rather than a problem to solve, the course of action would have been different.

Relationship Pole

The importance of this pole is most evident when changes result in positive outcomes, because focusing on relationships as well as productivity creates a team of colleagues connected by a shared purpose and meaning of the work. Colleagues work on building nurturing relationships and clarifying what each staff member needs to carry out his or her scope of practice and service effectively and efficiently. When there are healthy, partnering relationships between the team and the people they serve, there is a sense of belonging and of being a part of a supportive community of care. This enhances everyone's quality of life. The staff become collectively responsible for the cost, efficiency, and effectiveness of their care.

Action steps. Action steps to support this pole are essential. There will always be unexpected changes, increased demands, new challenges, and new barriers within the complex healthcare system. Having a foundational structure in place to deal with this reality *as a team* is critical because it brings the team together. Only if there is a place for the team to meet, engage in dialogue, and explore solutions together will innovative and creative possibilities emerge. Healthy relationships allow colleagues to honor one another's roles and value to the team. Accountability is basic to the necessary integration that stops duplication, repetition, and fragmentation of care and is an essential part of improving productivity. The work necessary to support the Relationships pole is actually a preventive measure taken to create a culture that is flexible enough to deal with changes and to innovate during a stressful period of fiscal instability. This clinic did not have that structure in place.

Those who favor or have job roles that are part of the Productivity pole have legitimate fears about the Relationships pole. They have seen the early warnings and downsides leading to lack of clarity regarding roles and lack of personal and collective responsibility for the work that needs to be accomplished to achieve effective, efficient, cost-effective care.

Clinical Scenario, continued:

The leadership in the clinic was clear that if there is "no margin," there will be "no mission." They knew that they had to increase productivity, but they failed to ask if it was a problem to solve or something that needed to be managed, or both. The fear that the walk-in clinic site might have to close made the manager more intense on the Productivity pole. The demand to decrease cost and enhance productivity is not going away. The Triple Aim clearly states the goal is to decrease the per capita cost of healthcare. No one argues the need to address this issue. It is how to make it happen.

The old way of thinking was that when there was a fiscal problem, there would be the usual problem-solving approach. This type of thinking puts those who give care as well as those who receive care at risk. Notice in the scenario that the problem approach was reflective of unilateral thinking related to the focus on the Vertical, Margin, Task, Directive Decision Making, and Project poles—and of course on the Productivity pole—to the neglect of the Horizontal, Mission, Scope of Practice, Shared Decision Making, Framework-Driven Change, and the Relationships poles.

It is important to remember that no matter how much time, money, and human resources are used, **if the problem is connected to a polarity and only one pole is focused on to the neglect of the other pole, the outcomes are predictable.**

Connecting a change process to an underlying polarity enhances the outcomes.

F. The Interprofessional Education and Collaborative Practice Polarity

The last polarity in this section is one that is challenging the whole of healthcare. Let's begin with what these two values are. Interprofessional Education refers to the learning that takes place between students from two or more professions in order to further collaborate and improve health outcomes. It is connected to sustainable integrated healthcare systems that stop duplication and repetition and deliver cost-effective, efficient, quality care.

Collaborative Practice refers to the work done by groups of healthcare workers from different professional backgrounds with patients, families, caregivers, and communities to deliver the highest quality of care possible—a level of care that would not be possible when a single homogeneous group works alone.

These two values hold the hope that we can improve healthcare today and create a better future for tomorrow. The education of our professionals and the extent to which we collaborate in practice are an interdependent pair, connected to every polarity that has been introduced in this book. As obvious as it is and as often as it is called for, we are not even close to achieving the upsides of both poles and the greater purpose that is possible for us. It is the Education and Practice polarity. More specifically it is the Interprofessional Education (IPE) and Collaborative Practice (CP) polarity.

This polarity is about you and me and the millions of our colleagues who at one point in our lives made a decision to become a healthcare professional. Some people refer to this calling as a decision to become a healer, but no matter what we call it, we have all dedicated our life's work to improving the health of this humanity.

We know that health will determine the quality of each person's life, and there are so many diverse ways in which we can make a difference. Each of us had to make a choice regarding how we would be able to make a difference. The obvious choices relate to those who provide care and prevent illness, such as nurses, the largest group; physicians with multiple specialties; psychologists; social workers; physical, respiratory, occupational, and speech therapists; dieticians; biometricians; pharmacists; technologists; environmentalists; academicians, researchers, etc.

No matter what the choice, we all began our journey by entering an education program. Our initial exposure to the profession takes place in a classroom where the theory related to the profession unfolds and at some point is enhanced by an introduction into the real world via simulations and clinical rotations. It is the combination of the two, theory and clinical experience, that forms our learning.

Why is the IPE/CP polarity getting so much attention? **The rising cost of health-care** concerns individuals, businesses, and of course the government. **Access to health-care** is also a problem for many people in our country. These are great challenges.

At the heart of the national call to improve quality care and lower costs was the realization that health outcomes are improved when the care is delivered by a team of professionals who work together to manage and deliver care. The national response to address these realities included several significant actions:

- In 2010, the World Health Organization identified interprofessional education and collaborative practice as an international necessity to prepare the future healthcare workforce to address local health needs.

- Implementation of the Affordable Care Act is driving changes in healthcare delivery to improve outcomes and lower costs, emphasizing interprofessional collaborative practice.

- In 2012, the U.S. Department of Health and Human Services designated the University of Minnesota as the National Center for Interprofessional Practice and Education.

- In 2013, the body that accredits all U.S. medical schools—the Liaison Committee on Medical Education—adopted a new accreditation standard mandating changes to the core curriculum of medical education programs in order to prepare medical students to be a part of collaborative teams that include other health professionals.

- The Accreditation Council for Pharmacy Education (ACPE) has implemented interprofessional education (IPE) standards.

- The American Association of Colleges of Nursing has integrated interprofessional collaboration and behavioral expectations into the "essentials" for baccalaureate, master's, and doctoral programs.

- The Institute of Medicine and the Interprofessional Education Collaborative have released interprofessional collaborative practice competencies to guide reform of health professions education.

With all this awareness and professional focus, why aren't the desired outcomes of this polarity being met? First of all many do not know this is a polarity, and action steps necessary to achieve the desired goals have not been implemented. In addition, this polarity calls for transformation of both Practice and Education. It requires intense work within two of the largest, bureaucratic cultures in our society: the healthcare system and the education system. It also calls for transformation of the whole acute care delivery model and the curriculum of hundreds of institutions of higher learning, including schools of nursing, medicine, pharmacy, and all allied curricula, such as curricula for physical, respiratory, occupational, and speech therapy programs, to name a few.

Let's take a look at a simple map that relates to IPE/CP in both settings. The one place where many of the healthcare disciplines come together is in the acute care setting, so we will use that lens for the Collaborative Practice pole.

We will use the education system context for preparing students for a professional career, using the acute care setting for their clinical exposure. The students (pre-licensure) will be the focus on the Interprofessonal Education pole, and the clinicians (post-licensure) will be the focus for the Collaborative Practice pole.

Completed Map for the Interprofessional Education and Collaborative Practice Polarity

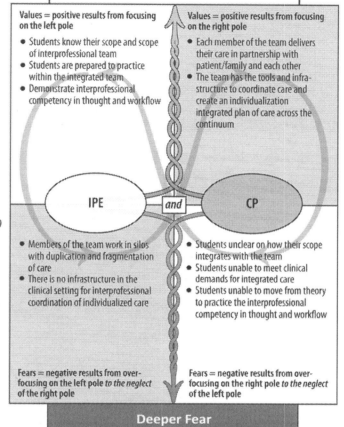

Greater Purpose Statement (GPS)
Efficient, effective integrated care
Why leverage this polarity?

Action Steps
How will we gain or maintain the positive results from focusing on this left pole? What? Who? By when? Measures?

A. Common vision for interprofessional education including faculty and curriculum education
B. Integration of core competencies for interprofessional practice and education into curriculum
C. Clarity on individual and team's scope of practice and overlap
D. Clinical and simulation experiences that provide knowledge and skills for inter-professional practice

Values = positive results from focusing on the left pole

- Students know their scope and scope of interprofessional team
- Students are prepared to practice within the integrated team
- Demonstrate interprofessional competency in thought and workflow

Values = positive results from focusing on the right pole

- Each member of the team delivers their care in partnership with patient/family and each other
- The team has the tools and infra-structure to coordinate care and create an individualization integrated plan of care across the continuum

Action Steps
How will we gain or maintain the positive results from focusing on this right pole? What? Who? By when? Measures?

A. Clarity on individual scope of practice
B. Clarity on team's scope of practice and overlap
C. Technology tools to support integrated competency, EMR functionality, EB guidelines of care, plan of care
D. Partnership infrastructure and skill development
E. Interprofessional documentation
F. Leveraging evidence-based integrated content

Early Warnings
Measurable indicators (things you can count) that will let you know that you are getting into the downside of this left pole.

A. Students upset that they never experience the theory in real world, complaining about teams they are on
B. "If IPE is so important, why don't we see it in the real world?"

IPE *and* CP

- Members of the team work in silos with duplication and fragmentation of care
- There is no infrastructure in the clinical setting for interprofessional coordination of individualized care

- Students unclear on how their scope integrates with the team
- Students unable to meet clinical demands for integrated care
- Students unable to move from theory to practice the interprofessional competency in thought and workflow

Early Warnings
Measurable indicators (things you can count) that will let you know that you are getting into the downside of this right pole.

A. Practitioners complaining students are interfering with the delivery of quality care
B. Practitioners complaining that students do not know how to work on a team
C. Students feel disrespected in clinical areas

Fears = negative results from over-focusing on the left pole *to the neglect* of the right pole

Fears = negative results from over-focusing on the right pole *to the neglect* of the left pole

Deeper Fear
Inefficient, ineffective, fragmented care
Loss of Greater Purpose

Reflections on the Interprofessional Education and Collaborative Practice Polarity

Upsides of the IPE pole. It is easy to identify with the upsides of the IPE pole, especially when it comes to students who are being prepared for the realities of clinical practice. The students will know their scope and the scope of practice for the interprofessional team members. The students will be prepared to practice within an integrated team. And the students can demonstrate competence in interprofessional-related thought and workflow.

What is interfering with these realistic and important outcomes? The action steps are where the problem sits. When a student comes into their profession, they are generally taught their scope of practice and are prepared to deliver it in the clinical setting. They are able to demonstrate the critical thinking necessary for their thought and workflow, but they are taught in isolation: their curriculum is specific only to their profession.

The IPE pole is calling for interprofessional education and integration, which now requires an additional accountability for all health profession faculties to take action steps, such as

- Have a common vision for interprofessional education that is reflected in their curriculum.
- Integrate core competencies for interprofessional practice and education into the curriculum.
- Achieve clarity on individual and team scope of practice and areas of overlap.
- Assure that clinical and simulation experiences provide knowledge and skills of integrated practice.

This all sounds good, but it requires extensive faculty and student preparation across multiple healthcare professions, which takes time, money, and resources. This work has not been done in most education settings, and the call for it to be done is coming at a time when the whole of the academic world is facing cost pressures, heavy faculty workloads, and less state and federal funding to support their institutions.

There are many areas that are important to the strengthening of this pole. One of these has to do with a fear that if IPE takes hold, the individual professions will lose their identity and be weakened. Many higher education faculty around the country already feel that there is not enough time within their curricula to teach the students their profession's unique scope of practice.

Upsides of the Collaborative Practice pole. Once again, it is easy to identify with the positive outcomes when this pole is supported. Each member of the team in the acute care setting is able to deliver care in partnership with the patient/family and one another, and the team has at its finger tips the tools and structural processes to coordinate care and create an individualized, integrated plan of care across the continuum.

As with all polarities, this Collaborative Practice pole must be backed up with strong action steps to achieve these outcomes. Once again, this is where the problem sits. These outcomes are critical if we intend to transform healthcare. The action steps on the map state that the members of the team will be clear about their individual as well as the team's scope of practice, and will know where there is overlap and how to integrate it. They will need technology tools to support integrated competency and functionality within the Electronic Health Record system that supports evidence-based guidelines, interprofessional documentation, and an integrated, individualized plan of care. Also important: a partnership foundational structure that brings the team together, as well as opportunities for team skill development.

There are acute care settings in this country that are doing this work. However, since most of the clinicians in these acute care settings have not been educated in IPE, the hospital setting needs to take on this education of their staff. In addition, it requires new tools and resources as well as a foundational infrastructure to make collaborative practice happen. At the same time there are major credentialing demands and payer reform at the state and national levels impacting every element of their financial stability. All of this is happening while they carry out their everyday practice and it takes time, money, and resources. Yet all of this needs to happen in order to have a Collaborative Practice setting for all healthcare providers.

Downsides of both poles. We already know the downsides of both poles because we are living them. Because IPE is not the norm in education, we still see students who are not clear about how their scope of practice integrates with the team, and we see students who are unable to meet clinical demands for integrated care and unable to integrate the theory of Interprofessional Competency in thought and workflow into their practice. The reason: No one has taught them these things.

We already know the downsides of neglecting the Collaborative Practice pole because we see clinicians working in so-called silos in many acute care settings and minimal use of foundational structures in the clinical settings for interprofessional coordination of individualized care because the organizations are not prepared for this type of practice and do not have tools to help them transition.

Early warnings. We see the early warnings as listed on the map. What is interesting and different from all the maps presented in this book is that the early warnings are limited to only those settings that are addressing one pole or the other.

For example, in one university, they are teaching IPE, but what do they hear from the students? They hear the early warning signs that students are upset because they never see the IPE theory being lived in their clinical rotations. They say, "If IPE is so important, why don't we see it in the real world?"

We see early warnings that are listed on the map for over-focusing on CP, but only from clinical settings where people are using the action steps to strengthen Collaborative Practice. The students who come to this clinical rotation often do not have an IPE background. You'll hear the clinicians in those settings saying things such as, "The students are interfering with the delivery of quality care." "They do not know how to work with the team." "The faculty will hear students saying that they are not feeling welcomed or that they feel disrespected in clinical areas because they are not meeting expectations."

What is missing? Both poles are being treated as a problem to solve by two different entities: education and the healthcare system. It is not the norm to have simultaneous dual accountability to create an integrated healthcare system by either the Education System or the Healthcare System. The leaders in these two entities have not identified this as a polarity and unless they come together to address this issue, we will not be able to reach or sustain an integrated healthcare system that is efficient, effective, and providing quality care for this humanity.

The downsides of this polarity map and the early warnings are the symptoms that this polarity is not being leveraged well. There is much work to be done. However, we know, the call and the need for it will continue because polarities don't go away. The awareness of the downsides are becoming stronger and stronger. Coupled with a greater awareness of polarities, we have much hope for the ability to reach the greater purpose in our future. That is why I end this section with this polarity because once it is visualized, we can count on our intelligent, committed colleagues to work on it, and over time, we will achieve our desired outcomes.

Polarity Thinking will speed up this process.

Section Two

Closing Thoughts

The Hope for Healthcare Transformation

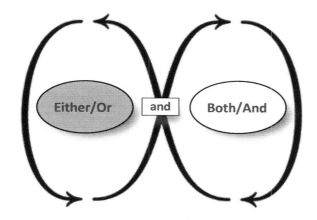

This book is a primer. There is much more to learn. Polarity Thinking is the missing logic needed in order to transform the healthcare system around the world. Those of us who have committed our professional lives to this work, coupled with our strong problem skills of *either/or* thinking and *both/and* Polarity Thinking, provide hope for reaching possibilities that most of us only hold in our hearts. *This book has described a new accountability for each of us. It is vigilance, essential to leverage the existing polarities.* It is a new expectation that breaks the bonds of complacency and moves our goals beyond fixing problems to creating new possibilities.

Can you imagine a healthcare system with cultures where we will no longer experience the downsides of any of the polarities we have reviewed in this book? I can imagine a healthcare system with cultures molded by the positive outcomes of each of the polarities not only in this book but those that surround us daily. Polarity Thinking is a reminder that we have the ability to know and enhance our reality and create our future.

We have learned in our work that many of the healthcare polarities not only relate to one another but impact each other. That is because they are all connected to the mission of healthcare, a mission that each of us committed to with our choice to be a part of the healthcare world. Since we are all experiencing many of the same polarities and we know they are not going away because they are unsolvable, unstoppable, and indestructible yet leverageable, we can help each other by sharing the action steps that help us achieve the greater purpose. We have a solid, tested approach and model for this new way of thinking. It is my hope you will use it to address the paradoxes that surround you every day and help you reach the goals, the greater purpose you hold in your heart.

William Butler Yeats said, "Education is not the filling of a pail, but the lighting of a fire." I hope this book helps light the fire in your belly about Polarity Thinking.

Polarity Thinking

We need to know self
But cannot unless we know who we are with others.
We can disconnect and become paralyzed with divergent thinking
But without Polarity Thinking we become paralyzed in old ways.
Creating collective thinking is essential
But individuals must stay true to the voice of their soul.
We must be a team
But the team is weak without strong individuals.
We must create an integrated healthcare system
But each part must be self-sufficient and effective.
There is no margin without mission
But there is no mission without margin.
We must collectively be certain what matters most
But first we must unmask personal certainty.
Positive energy ignites action
But negative energy also ignites action.
Our passion can provoke the action of others
But our passion can suffocate the fire of another's passion.
We transcend polarities when we connect at the soul
The soul holds no polarities, only greater purpose.

— Bonnie Wesorick

If you would like further information, please contact the Interprofessional Institute for Polarity Thinking in Healthcare located at Grand Valley State University. gvsu@edu.com

Section Three:
Summary of Principles, Tips, and Strategies

Section Three

Summary of Principles, Tips, and Strategies

There are many principles, key statements and perspectives throughout this book. The following summary is provided to give a brief review to facilitate the recall of fundamental elements related to the whole of Polarity Thinking.

- Today's healthcare leaders are responsible to accurately diagnose the reality that surrounds them. Misdiagnosis of reality puts both those who give and receive care at risk. Polarity Thinking is a skill that provides insights into the complex reality of healthcare, giving hope and direction to improve reality.

- Polarities are interdependent pairs of values or alternative points of view that are different and may appear as unrelated, competitive, or opposite, but need each other over time to reach outcomes that neither could reach alone. They are often called dilemmas, paradoxes, or chronic issues. Each value only represents half of the truth. It is foreign to think of opposite as connected or interdependent.

- When leaders misdiagnose a polarity for a problem, there are unintended consequences for both those who give and receive care. When leaders are not clear about how to differentiate between problems and polarities, there is wasted time, money, and energy.

- Polarity Thinking is a supplement to problem solving not a replacement and can be visualized via a polarity map.

- The basic polarity map has 11 components: each component of the pair is called a pole, an infinity loop representing the reality of the tension/energy dynamics between the poles, four quadrants (one for placement of the positive and negative outcomes of each pole), two arrows representing the synergy between quadrants (one virtuous leading to the greater purpose component and one vicious leading to the deeper fear/concern component).

- Interdependent poles should have value neutral names or valued positive names. If one is positive and the other is negative, it will look like a problem to solve. Both poles have positive outcomes or an "upside" as well as "downsides" or negative outcomes.

- One pole of a polarity represents two parts of the map: the positive value and the fear of loss of the positive value are placed on the map in a diagonal quadrant. The true opposites within a polarity are the diagonal quadrants.

- There is 100% predictability that there will be negative outcomes if one pole is neglected. You will first get the downside of the very pole you are concentrating on. Overtime you will also get the downside of the other pole. Most symptoms of the downside of a pole are not evident right away.

- Polarities never go away; they are not problems to be solved. They are unavoidable, unsolvable, indestructible, but most important leverageable.

- Since one pole of a polarity is unsustainable, tying a change effort to one pole of a polarity will make the change effort unsustainable. Tying a change effort to both poles of a polarity increases attainability and sustainability because polarities are indestructible.

- A virtuous cycle is created when the energy/tension between both upsides is leveraged, leading to outcomes unattainable by either pole alone. This outcome is called the greater purpose. The greater purpose answers the question, "Why bother to manage the polarity well?" It is an answer that works for both those preferring the left pole and those preferring the right pole.

- Oscillation prevents getting stuck in the downside of one pole or the other. It also helps avoid the extreme downsides of either pole. Oscillation is less obvious when there are enough people dedicated to support each pole. With simultaneous support of both poles, the positive outcomes, not the swinging effect, are sustainable because the tension between the poles is being leveraged to catapult to a higher purpose.

- Excellent practitioners and leaders are master problem solvers. Problem solving calls for *either/or* thinking and Polarity Thinking calls for *both/and* thinking. *Both are essential.* Polarity Thinking is not a replacement for *either/or* thinking; it is a supplement. One of the major differences between problem solving and Polarity Thinking is the demand for continuous vigilance to leverage the polarity.

- If you misdiagnose any polarity as a problem to be solved, you will over time, always be unsuccessful. Having a common model and set of principles makes it easier to intentionally work with others to tap the huge potential when polarities are leveraged. Overall the goal is to be both proactive (ensure each pole is supported) and reactive (ensure that one pole is not focused on at the neglect of the other).

- Action steps list the interventions necessary to maintain and sustain the desired outcomes of the pole. The action steps keep the energy flow between the poles moving in a virtuous fashion leading to the greater purpose. Sometimes it is easier to list interventions to strengthen your preference pole rather than to list interventions for the opposite pole.

- Early warnings ensure that one pole does not get focused on at the neglect of the other pole and help us prevent slipping back into our problem-solving mode of thinking. They are measurable and act as early indicators that you are getting into the downside of a pole.

- It is important to know which pole is your preference, no matter how subtle it is. Remember if you are a person in a power position, the people around you may be living in the downside of your pole preference. The downside of one's preference pole is difficult to describe; it is your blind spot.

- The concept of "over time" is an important principle of polarities. The clearer you communicate your point of view as a problem and logical solution, the greater the resistance from those holding the alternative point of view. The weaker your opposition, the more you need to listen.

- When starting to fill in a map, start with the person's preferred pole. This assures them it will be honored. It is then easier for them to explore the opposite values.

- Often there is no quick fix for polarities; there are short- and long-term strategies to leverage the tension/energy between the poles.

- Polarity Thinking prevents the pendulum effect associated with focus on one pole as a problem to solve and then focus on the other as a problem to solve.

- The first question to be asked anytime there is a situation of concern brought up: Is this a problem to be solved or a polarity to be leveraged or both? If a polarity is seen as a problem, any effort will generate its own resistance, have a reduced chance of attaining a goal, and even if the goal is being experienced, it will be done slower than necessary and it will be unsustainable over time.

- It is natural to resist any change effort that does not acknowledge the opposite polarity no matter how important the idea is. When people see what they value being supported and the desire to prevent the downside of the opposite pole, it takes away the need to resist. The normal tension/ energy between poles can be seen as resistance. Resistance will always be present if a person is living in the downside of the very pole that is being focused on.

- The stronger you believe that the change is going to fix the problem, the stronger you believe that those who resist it are wrong. This increases conflict. If the polarity is being handled as a problem to solve, it is worse than a waste of time; it is destructive, which means you pay twice. When polarities are leveraged well, the resistance is leveraged and becomes a resource to catapult to a greater purpose, which is something both poles value.

- Polarities show up in three ways: conflicts, complaints, and/or resistance to change. If a polarity is misdiagnosed as a problem to be solved, it is 100% predictable that the change effort will fail over time and costly efforts will be wasted. Misdiagnosed change efforts can attain some positive out-comes for a while, but these outcomes will not be sustainable over time.

- The stronger your value for one pole, the harder it is to know or recognize your preference pole's downside. The stronger and longer one has experienced living in the downside of a dominant pole, the greater the resistance to any focus on supporting that pole. The stronger one values the upside of one pole, the greater will be the fear of the downside of the opposite pole. Thus, even though we may intellectually agree with the need to shift to the upside of the opposite pole, we may resist going there because of the fear of the downside of the opposite pole. This keeps us from "walking our talk."

- We often make our promises from our deep values, but our actions are more a reflection of our fears. When people see what they value being supported and the desire to prevent the downside of the opposite pole, it takes away the need to resist.

- Because of our *either/or* thinking, the most natural thing is to try and get others to think like you. It is rare to reach out and encourage others to stay strong in their opposing view. Polarity Thinking helps you do that. It is never about choosing one pole or the other. It is about the need to embrace both poles and the tension between them. With all polarities, it is win/win.

- The Project/Framework polarity (Part/Whole) is new to healthcare. The Part (Project) is strong, but the Framework pole (Whole) is new. The Complexity of the healthcare system requires a Framework to guide action steps necessary to reach the greater purpose. The Framework pole pre-vents going to the downside of the Project pole. When there is an understanding that each project relates to a greater whole, it brings the action steps to a different level.

- The polarity map takes the invisible truths about the power of leadership and makes them visible. Leaders who manage polarities know how to remove fear from the work culture. Relationship polarities are the mother of all polarities.

- When power becomes "power over," no polarity can be leveraged. When a person is imposing his/ her pole, he/she does not feel the tension. Polarity allows you to hang onto or hold true to your view but also see the truth of the opposite view and together learn how to do both.

- Polarity Thinking eliminates the paralysis of fear and creates an oscillation that leverages the situa-tion so that we know how to ensure that the legitimate fears of the downsides do not become reality.

- The call to automate is very different from the call to transform culture and practice using technology.

- The EHR relates to a major polarity for healthcare leaders: Technology Platform/Practice Platform polarity.

- Leveraging polarities is fundamental to achieve exponential growth.

- When a mandate is known to be a polarity, the approach, action steps, and direction of many organizations will be different.

- The gift of polarities is that it helps you see that you no longer have to live a life divided. Polarity Thinking allows you to hang onto or hold true to your view but also see the truth of the opposite view and learn how together these values can reach a goal neither can do alone.

- Polarity Thinking takes away the unnecessary use of energy spent on trying to convince everyone else to think like you do.

- The methods and metrics that address problem solving are insufficient for evaluating how well the organization is leveraging polarities. New tools demonstrate real time feedback on the status of efforts to leverage polarities.

- Too much time, money, and energy have been wasted, and lasting success has remained elusive when leaders have focused on fixing broken things instead of understanding the underlying cause of issues in the organization.

Bibliography

Ackoff, R. (1986). *Management in small doses*. New York: John Wiley and Sons.

Abrahamson K., Arling P., Wesorick B., & Anderson J. (2012, January–March). An application of the socio technical systems approach to implementation of electronic evidence into practice: The Clinical Practice Model framework. *International Journal of Reliable and Quality E Healthcare, 1*(1), 13–20.

AHRQ (2008). Hospital survey on patient safety culture. Comparison Data Base Reports. Retrieved May 2010 from http://www.ahrq.gov/qual/hospsurvey08/

Berwick, D., & Hackbarth, A. D. (2012). Eliminating waste in U.S. healthcare. *JAMA, 307*(14), 1513–1516.

Blumenthal, D. (2009). Stimulating the adoption of health information technology. *The New England Journal of Medicine, 260*(15), 1376–1479.

Blumenthal, D. (2014). Realizing the rewards of a medical career in a changing healthcare system. Speech at the 2014 Columbia University College of Physicians and Surgeons graduation ceremony.

Bowman, S. (2013, Fall). Impact of electronic health record systems on information integrity: Quality and safety implications. *Perspectives in Health Information Management,* 1–18.

Center for Creative Leadership. (2013). *Leading Effectively e-Newsletter*. Greensboro, North Carolina.

Christopherson, T. (2011, November). The electronic health record: Implications for interprofessional education and practice. Paper presented at the meeting of the Collaborating Across Borders III Conference, Tucson, Arizona.

Classen, D., Lloyd, R., Provost, L., Griffin, F., & Resar, R. (2008). Development and evaluation of the institute for healthcare improvement global trigger tool. *Journal of Patient Safety, 4*(3).

Classen, D., Resar, R., Griffin, F., Federico, R., Frankel T., Kimmel N., Whittington J., Frankel, A., Seger, A., & Brent, J. (2011). Global trigger tool shows that adverse events in hospitals may be 10 times greater than previously measured. *Health Affairs, 30*(4), 1–9.

Collins, J. D., & Porras, J. I. (1994). *Built to last: successful habits of visionary companies*. New York: Harper Collins.

Collins, J. (2001). Good to great: Why some companies make the leap and others don't. New York: Harper Collins.

Commonwealth Fund. (2014). Mirror, Mirror on the Wall, 2014 Update: How the U.S. Healthcare System Compares Internationally. http://www.commonwealthfund. Org/publications/fund-reports/2014/june/mirror-mirror. Covey, S.R. (1992). *Principle-centered leadership*. New York: Simon and Schuster.

Covey, S.R. (1990). *The 7 habits of highly effective people: Powerful lessons in personal change*. New York: Simon and Schuster.

De Pree, M. (1989). *Leadership is an Art*. New York: Doubleday.

Devitt, B., & Meyer, R. (1999). *Strategy synthesis: Resolving strategy paradoxes to create competitive advantage*. London: Thompson.

Dodd, D., & Favaro, K. (2007). *The three tensions: Winning the struggle to perform without compromise*. New York: Wiley and Sons.

Elsevier CPM Resource Center (2011). The CPM Framework™: Culture and professional practice for sustainable healthcare transformation. (Brochure). Grand Rapids, MI.

Elsevier CPM International Consortium Summit Proceedings (2009). Grand Rapids, MI.

Elsner, R. & Farrands, B. (2006). *Lost in transition: How business leaders can successfully take charge in new roles.* London: Marshall Cavendish Limited.

Felt-Lists, Ferry, G., Rober, R., AuM, Walker, J., Jones, J.B., & Lerch S. (December 2012). *Sustainability, partnerships and teamwork in health IT implementation: Essential finding from the transforming healthcare quality through IT* grant. AHRQ Publication. Rockville, MD: Agency for Healthcare Research and Quality.

Fletcher, J., & Olwyler, K. (1997). *Paradoxical thinking: How to profit from your contradictions.* San Francisco, CA: Berrett-Koehler.

Gebbie, K., Rosenstock, L., & Hernandez, L.M. (Eds.) (2003). *Who will keep the public healthy? Educating public health professionals for the 21st century.* Washington, DC: The National Academies Press.

Hanson, D., Hoss, B. L., Wesorick, B. (2008). Evaluating the evidence: Guidelines. *AORN Journal, 88*, 184–195.

Hanson, D. (2011). Evidence-based clinical decision support. In M. J. Ball & K. J. Hannah (Eds.). *Nursing informatics: Where technology and caring meet* (4), 243–258. New York: Springer.

Institute for Healthcare Improvement (IHI). Triple Aim. Retrieved December 2011 from http://www.ihi.org

Institute of Medicine. (2001). *Crossing the quality chasm: A new health system for the 21st century.* Committee on Quality of Healthcare in America. Washington, DC: National Academies Press.

Institute of Medicine. (2003). *Keeping patients safe: Transforming the work environment of nurses.* Committee of the Work Environment for Nurses and Patient Safety. Washington, DC: National Academies Press.

Institute of Medicine Report. (2003). *Health professions education: A bridge to quality.* Washington, DC National Academies Press.

Institute of Medicine. (2011). *Digital infrastructure for the learning health system: The foundation for continuous improvement in health and healthcare.* Washington, DC: National Academies Press.

Institute of Medicine. (2011). *Health IT and patient safety: Building safer systems for better care.* Washington, DC: National Academies Press.

Institute of Medicine. (2012). *Best care at lower cost.* Washington, DC: National Academies Press.

Institute of Medicine. (2014). *Capturing social and behavioral domains in electronic health records: Phase 1.* Washington, DC; National Academies Press.

Interprofessional Education Collaborative Expert Panel. (2011). Core competencies for interprofessional collaborative practice: Report of an expert panel. Washington, DC: Interprofessional Education Collaborative, p. 9.

Johnson, B. (1992, 1996). *Polarity management: Identifying and managing unsolvable problems.* Amherst, MA: HRD Press, Inc.

Kenny, C. (2008). *The best practice: How the new quality movement is transforming medicine.* New York: Public Affairs.

Kohn, L. T., Corrigan, J. M., & Donaldson, M. S., (Eds). (1999). *To err is human: Building a safer health system.* Washington, DC: National Academies Press.

Mason, J., & Wesorick, B. (2011). Successful transformation of a nursing culture. *Nurse Leader, 9*(2), 31–36.

McGrath, R. (2012). How growth outliers do it. *Harvard Business Review, 90*(1), 110–116.

National Quality Forum (NQF). (2010). Safe practices for better healthcare—2010 Update: A consensus report. Washington, DC: NQF.

Naisbett, J. (2006). *Mind Set! Reset your thinking and see the future*. New York: Harper Collins Publisher.

Oswald, R., & Johnson, B. (2009). *Managing polarities in congregations: Eight keys for thriving communities*. Amherst, MA: HRD Press.

Reid, T. R. (2010). *The healing of America: A global quest for better, cheaper, and fairer healthcare*. New York: Penguin Books.

Seidler, M. (2008). *Power surge: A conduit for enlightened leadership*. Amherst, MA: HRD Press.

Staggers N., & Troseth, M. (2011). The role of usability and clinical application design in health information technology adoption. *Nursing Informatics*. In M. Ball, et al., Eds. *Nursing Informatics: Where Caring and Technology Meet* (4th ed.). New York: Springer Publishing.

The Joint Commission. (2012). *2012 hospital accreditation standards: Provision of care, treatment, and services (PC.02.02.01, PC.04.02.01)*. Oakbrook, IL: The Joint Commission. Retrieved January 2012 from http://www.jointcommission.org

The Tiger Initiative Foundation. (2014). The Leadership Imperative: Tiger's Recommendations for Integrating Technology to Transform Practice and Education. http://www.thetigerinitiative.org/

Wesorick, B., & Doebbeling, B. (2011). Lessons from the field: The essential elements for point-of-care transformation. *Medical Care, 49*(12), Suppl 1, S49–S58.

Wesorick, B., Troseth, M., & Cato, J. (2004). Intentionally designed automation creates the best places to work and receive care. In *Health care technology: Innovating care through technology*, 2. San Francisco, CA: Montgomery Research, Inc.

Wesorick, B. (2002). 21st century leadership challenge: Creating and sustaining healthy, healing work cultures and integrated service at the point of care. *Nursing Administration Quarterly, 26*(5), 18–32.

Wesorick, B., Shiparski, L., Troseth, M., et al. (1998). *Partnership Council field book: Strategies and tools for co-creating a health work place*. Grand Rapids, MI: Practice Field Publishing.

Wesorick, B. (2008). Live a legacy or live a lie. *Nursing Administration Quarterly, 32*(2), 142–158.

Wesorick, B. (2013). Essential steps for successful implementation of the EHR to achieve sustainable, safe, quality care. In A. Moumtzoglou & A. Katrinia. *E-Health technologies and improving patient safety: Exposing organizational factors. Hershey*, PA: IGI Global, p. 27–55.

Wesorick, B. (2014). Polarity thinking: An essential skill for those leading interprofessional integration, *Journal of Interprofessional Healthcare 1*(1), Article 12.